THE NEXT CHAPTER
ESSL:
EARLY SCREENING SAVES LIVES

"AMBASSADOR" JOE GREENE

THE BLACK SPOKESMAN FOR COLONOSCOPY TESTING AT AGE 40

This is dedicated to my kids, my nieces, and my nephews.

Remember your Daddy and Uncle is a Fighter

and will NEVER GIVE UP.

ESSL

Early Screening Saves Lives

Asheville, NC

Cover Design: Dorian Harris, The Art Dealer, Inc.

Publishing Consultant: Sedrik Newbern, Newbern Consulting, LLC

Editor: Linda Shew Wolf, Network Publishing Partners, Inc.

Printed in the United States of America
First Edition: March 2023

ISBN Paperback: 979-8-218-17698-3
Library of Congress Control Number: 2023905957

Images:
Gastrointestinal anatomy. © 2017 American Cancer Society. Used with permission.
Colon anatomy. © 2017 American Cancer Society. Used with permission.

Disclaimer:
This book is designed to provide information in regard to the subject matter covered. It is sold with the understanding that the publisher and author are not engaged in rendering medical, naturopathic, homeopathic or other professional services. If medical or other expert assistance is required, the services of a competent professional should be sought. Every effort has been made to make this book as complete and accurate as possible. However, there may be mistakes both typographical and in content. Therefore this book should be used only as a general guide and not as the ultimate source of information on intestinal health. Furthermore, this book contains information only up to the printing date. The purpose of this book is to educate and entertain. The author and publisher shall have neither liability nor responsibility to any person or entity with respect to any loss or damage caused, or alleged to be caused, directly or indirectly by the information contained in this book.

Table of Contents

INTRODUCTION: TO MY COMMUNITY

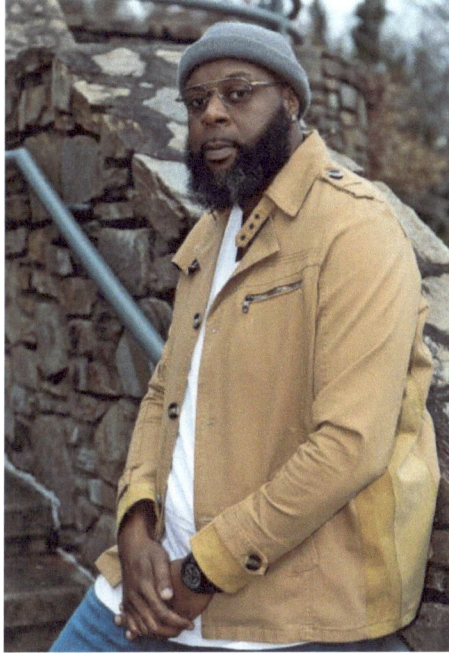

Chadwick Boseman, the star of *Black Panther*, died from colon cancer at age 43. After that, the covered age for a colonoscopy was reduced from 50 to 45. It may not have been just because of his death, but I think it had something to do with it. The mortality numbers in Black communities are on the rise.

I'm fighting to get the age lowered to 40 for starters. And I hope we can get the age below 40, because nurses and doctors are telling me that in the last two years with Covid, the rates of colon cancer for people aged 30 and under are up 75%. Up 75%! This is about everybody, but the Black community has the highest rate of all.

INTRODUCTION

If you have insurance, it won't cover the test below age 45 even if you have symptoms. The fact is, a lot of us in the Black community won't even see 45. This is a conversation that has never occurred in our community, and it must take place.

Black males and females have the highest incidence and mortality with colon cancer. The numbers are higher than whites, American Indians, Alaskan Natives, and Pacific Islanders. African Americans are about 20% more likely to be diagnosed with colon cancer and about 40% more likely to die from it than any other groups. Collectively Blacks have the shortest survival of any racial/ethnic group.

As a Black man, I know all about toughing things out and avoiding the doctor. It's typical behavior for us, but it's time to wake up to this danger. In my case, I was only 40 when I acknowledged to myself that something was wrong, but I really started wondering about it long before age 40. If you feel something isn't right, you can't just ignore it or chalk it up to aging or your imagination. There are more and more cases of intestinal cancer in people under 30 years old.

In my case, I was only 40 when I finally stopped putting off a colonoscopy. It's a good thing I woke up to it at last, because I was already pretty far gone. The drastic surgery and treatments I've been through saved my life, but they could have been avoided if I'd had a colonoscopy earlier. I'm a father first, and I'm now going through the challenges and fears of living with Stage 3 colon cancer. I'm not letting it knock me down or get in the way of quality time with my kids – just taking the good with the bad, and making it something it's supposed to be.

I don't want this to happen to anyone else, so I'm going to give you all the details, holding nothing back, so you can know what to expect during each step of the colon cancer journey. You will see signs if something is wrong, and you know your own body. If you feel that something is different and isn't going right, you need to get checked. That's why I am writing this book, and it's why I started ESSL, Early Screening Saves Lives.

My goal is to put pressure on policymakers to make colonoscopies at age 40 routinely covered by all insurance carriers. I'm thankful to be here, and I'm going to keep fighting. I'm the Black spokesman for colonoscopy testing at age 40.

My hope and prayer is that reading this book will inspire you to become aware, get tested, and stay ahead of this disease that is killing people in record numbers, especially men or color. I tell everyone who will listen, "This ain't nothing I heard . . . THIS IS WHAT I'M LIVING! F-cancer, keep it pushing. No need to complain – I have no time for that."

Let's fix this. Early Screening Saves Lives!

CHAPTER 1

AWARENESS

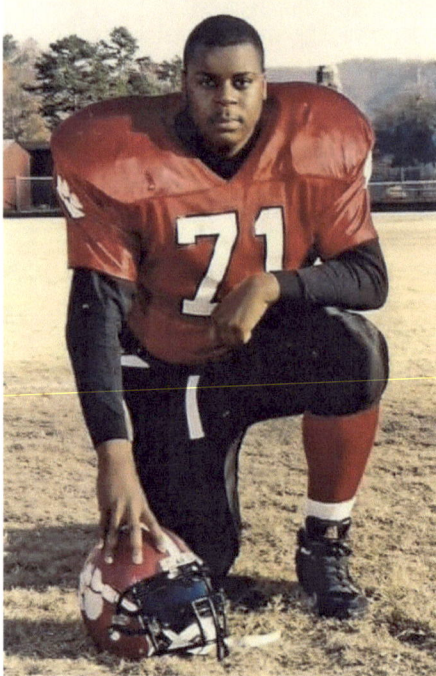

How would you feel if doctors told you that you have cancer, and not only that, that you were just weeks away from NOT being able to take a shit, ever again, without emergency surgery?

I couldn't wrap my head around that news. I never thought anything like this would ever happen to me. I still can't accept it to this day. Growing up, I had no reason to suspect anything would go wrong with my body. At least not something like this!

I have been living in Asheville, North Carolina nearly all my life. As a kid, I was fortunate to have a two-parent home with my brother and two sisters. We gained a lot of strength from our parents. I'm not saying everything was always perfect, but it was life. It was a full life.

My siblings and I are still together and close. My parents and my little sister live nearby, and my other siblings live in Concord and Huntersville. My Uncle Michael who watched over me growing up lives in Georgia, but we are all full of love and support for each other — so important. None of my siblings have any challenges with their health. They're going through life changes for sure, but as for cancer and other diseases, I'm thankful that they don't have to live through this. Doctors told me that my colon cancer is nothing that was passed down to me genetically. Nobody in my family line has had colon cancer before. I'm the first.

My parents were my main mentors growing up. Mama was a nurse back when Mission Hospital was called St. Joseph's. She was up on the 4th floor. She also worked at a rehabilitation center at some point when I was young. Sometimes, my siblings and I had to stay the night with her while she was on the night shift there if she didn't have childcare coverage. I remember the chocolate milk and graham crackers and especially the tiny containers of ice cream. Even with those perks, though, I complained to Mama about having to stay there when she came in to check on us.

"Why don't you like it, Joe?" she asked me. "They're so nice to you all. You get all these delicious treats and you sleep in this beautiful, quiet Physical Therapy room."

"But Mom, it smells bad in here!" I replied, holding my nose. She just laughed at me and waved me away back to my bed. I credit this as the beginning of my distaste for medical facilities.

By the time I was a teenager, though, medical facilities became a big part of our family's life. Mama developed symptoms that seemed to mystify her doctors. Looking back, I have to wonder how seriously they were listening to her. She ended up pushing for a diagnosis and not accepting the one being told to her. Being her own advocate and informing her GYN doctor of her symptoms and concerns was the pivot point for future testing which confirmed her ovarian cancer, Stage 2. She was right, there was something wrong.

I drove her to medical appointments, chemotherapy sessions, and biweekly follow-up tests after her chemotherapy. I remember driving her every other Monday from 8 to 4 to chemo. She was sensitive to the medications and would have reactions during testing and treatments, so it wasn't an easy road for her. When Mama was going through her cancer treatments it was like an out-of-body experience to me. As I drove her to many of her treatments, I would look over at her as she rested in the seat next to me. She looked so vulnerable.

It wasn't hard to be strong for her because I needed and wanted to be strong for my Mama. She was emotional and sad when she lost her long, beautiful hair. I couldn't relate at the time, but now I can. I didn't get it, the loss of your identity. The feelings of having no control over what was happening with your body, the medication, the port in your chest, the weakness and then the loss of the only thing you feel control over . . . your hair.

But she was strong about the whole thing – losing her hair, and all the exhaustion, nausea, and discomfort. I will never forget how powerful she was and how she insisted on keeping a positive outlook no matter what she was going through.

"Mama, how are you doing now?" I would ask her as we drove home from a chemo session or a test. I could see that she was sick to her stomach. Sometimes her hand would grip the seat belt just over her waist to keep it from pressing on her stomach, and I felt bad for her.

"Joe, I'm doing as good as anyone can expect," she would say. "Now, I want to hear all about your football practice yesterday." And we would drive home just talking about normal everyday things. After her long battle, she made it through all her treatments, surgeries, and tests to beat the cancer.

Not only was Mama going through a challenging time with her health, but my father's kidney disease was getting worse and worse. Around the time Mama's treatments were ending, Dad had to go on dialysis for about 5 or 6 years. I would drive him to dialysis at 6 a.m. every Monday, Wednesday, and Friday. While he was there having his treatment, if it was a chemo Monday for Mama, I would go back to get her to her treatment at 8 a.m., then go pick up Dad at noon and make sure he had lunch after his dialysis session.

I paid close attention to how Dad handled his life-threatening disease. He was always steady and reasonable. Just like Mama, he didn't want to talk about his feelings or dwell on his pain. I knew he was fighting not just for himself but for us. When he finally had a kidney transplant, it went very well and he's still him. He's still here with us.

Going through all this with both parents, I was aware that health could be fragile and medical problems could be dangerous. Like most young people leaving high school and heading out to college and work, though, I believed that I was invincible and that my body would never do that to me. I counted on that.

I was very excited to be playing football at North Carolina A&T in Greensboro, NC (GHOE). I practiced hard, played hard, studied hard, and lived life to the fullest. It was a very physically demanding time. Both my parents had conquered their illnesses, and now I was on my own, forging my own way forward. I wasn't going to let anything slow me down.

CHAPTER 2

AVOIDANCE

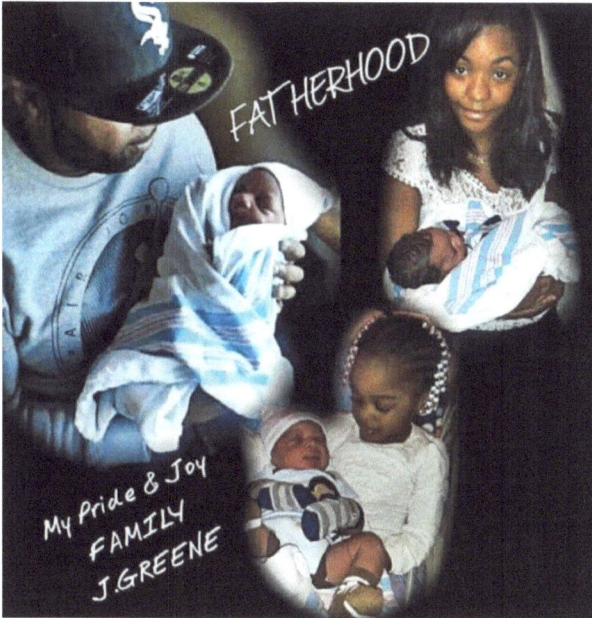

The first sign of trouble was not one I had much patience for. In 1999, I left for college and I ended up having my first GI series with barium in 2000. I had to come back to Asheville to get the test done. I had lost 30 pounds during my sophomore season and was throwing up a lot. There was a lot of acid in my stomach that burned a lot coming up, and even though I kept up the same level of exertion with football and studies, it affected my appetite after a while.

All through college, I ate whatever I wanted to eat, slept however little or much I felt like sleeping, and couldn't really accept that anything would ever go wrong with my body. Not knowing about stress, I didn't make the connection between my diet, my sleep schedule, and my health. When they found so much acid in my stomach, the doctors said I could use over-the-counter medicines to reduce it.

"Okay," I said. I tried a few acid reducers and found that Zantac worked the best. I had to take it often at first, but then I could get by with just one. If you look up Zantac now, the first thing that comes up is Zantac and cancer. I took Zantac for a little over 15 years straight.

I had been feeling that something wasn't normal for years before my cancer diagnosis, but I chose to push it to the side over and over again. I would just deal with it at another moment in time, I told myself. This was becoming more and more of a typical occurrence as each year rolled by. After I ate something, I would feel full.

My stomach felt bloated and I could feel the pressure of stool that wouldn't come out. I felt it all the way from my stomach to my butt hole. I'd be sitting on the toilet thinking, "How long have I been here?" The time would just drag. My leg would be falling asleep while my mind raced ahead to things I needed to do, and all the while, I was pushing and straining.

I was getting so tired of this same old, same old. When I couldn't stand the waiting anymore, I would make a stronger effort. When I felt it finally starting to move, then it would stop. It would just stop! Can you imagine how mind-blowing this whole thing is? You're sitting on the toilet, trying to get some kind of relief. Finally, you feel something moving down, but when you stand up, there is nothing. Damn. And there you go sitting down again to wait and try again and again, wishing and hoping just to be done.

The mental anguish, the denial that something was wrong, and the pride I felt as a man that required me to tough it out – this all led to my decision to ignore the problems I was having just trying to take a shit, which should be a regular process for a man to do.

One day, I went to the store to get some more Zantac because I had heartburn, and it was gone. It wasn't anywhere in the store for me to buy. I waited about a week or so and went back to the same store to get it and it was still gone. So, I called Mama to see if she could find it at another store, and she couldn't find it either.

Turns out, they had pulled it off the shelves worldwide because it was causing cancer in people's bodies. I'm not saying that's the reason for my cancer, and I'm not saying it's not the reason. I don't know for sure yet, but it's something I've been looking into. I went on the Zantac website and applied for compensation, but I haven't gotten any response yet.

AVOIDANCE

Later, after my surgery and treatments, my cancer doctor talked to me about genetic testing and its importance. It provides information on whether you carry the mutated gene and inherited a high risk for colorectal cancer which would run in your family. Genetic testing and knowing your family history can be instrumental in being aware of symptoms and guiding you toward screening, cancer prevention, and treatment plans. This testing can help prepare your family for their future with conversations and being open about our family histories around diagnoses such as colon cancer.

By having a genetic test, I learned the cancer was not genetically in my bloodline; the results were not hereditary. But because I was diagnosed at such a young age, the recommendation for early screening for my children and my continued bloodline can be the difference in preventative care or being diagnosed with colon cancer. Could it have been the Zantac, the environment, the food we eat, or all three? Either way, I applied to Zantac.

All those years, my whole mission was just to get the acid in my stomach down – I never thought anything about cancer.

After college, things started to get more challenging. Since I was having so much trouble using the restroom, I stopped eating red meat because it wasn't breaking down in my body anymore. I could feel it just sitting there, making it even harder to go. I was finally starting to listen to my body.

People think it's funny if they break wind and say, "Ooh that stinks!" I used to laugh right along with them. But really, that smell is something in your body breeding bacteria and living a life of its own. I'm not saying we all have to run out there and be extra healthy in all our choices, but when things change, it's time to pay attention to what's going on.

The more I stopped eating red meat, the more I started seeing how my body changed for the better. Even with this change for the better in my diet, my digestion was still sluggish and uncomfortable. I just thought it was because I was getting older. That was my mindset. This was just a natural part of getting a little older. No big deal.

The whole time something wasn't right.

I wasn't weak or tired. I was still walking every day and keeping myself in shape. I was in my 30s, so I wasn't training for football or staying as active physically. I had seen a post years before about 30-minute walks and what they do for you. So I started doing 30-minute walks in my neighborhood. I didn't go far. It helps relieve stress and it helps you lose weight, so I started a Facebook challenge for family and friends and built a fan base to get others to do it, too. It's just healthy for everyone. Since I couldn't run around several blocks like I used to, I had to find a way to get out there and get the blood flowing, somehow, some way.

AVOIDANCE

In my 30s, I was an entrepreneur with a couple of businesses. I was into nightlife entertainment producing parties, shows, concerts, and all kinds of events. I had a record label called Southern Boy Entertainment with Big Dreek and other hip-hop and R&B artists. I ran a club in Charlotte, running all the events.

It was a wild time and packed with good people, excitement, and learning experiences about how to be on my own. I also am a part owner of two barbershops in Charlotte called "No Grease" at Northlake Mall and "No Grease Premium" in Charlotte Premium Outlets. In addition, I launched a clothing line called BigBoiFly for big dudes who say they can't find clothes to fit them.

I was working in Charlotte and living in Asheville, so I traveled back and forth on the road a lot. I was starting to notice my bathroom problems more and more, like my body wasn't really breaking down food the same way. But we keep going on with life, we as men, we aren't really taking too much heed. I just kept telling myself, "Okay, whatever, it'll be all right."

You know how it goes – you don't really see your primary doctor more than once a year, and then it's only for 30 minutes max. They're not going to sit all day with you. They'll ask you what's going on with you, you'll tell them, and they'll give you the best solution they can give you, then on to the next patient.

It typically went like this:

"Doc, I still can't go to the toilet like I need to. I changed my diet. Well, I tried to. I'm eating more vegetables when I can, and I cut way back on eating red meat, but it seems to be getting harder and harder to break the food down."

This conversation was repeated over the course of a few years before I was diagnosed. It became more intense each year:

"Damn, Doc, it's getting harder and harder. Despite all the changes I have made, I still have to push and strain and now it's all the time with little and sometimes no results."

We would come up with the same plans . . . more roughage in my diet, taking stool softeners, drinking more water. By this time I had eliminated red meat from my diet, kept up the walks around my neighborhood every day for 30 minutes, and had lost a lot of weight. I honestly thought my weight loss was from all the walking and my changed diet. Looking back, I don't remember the word "cancer" coming up in any of our conversations or hearing a doctor question me about anyone in my family having a history of colon cancer.

Maybe because of my age, I considered myself to be a healthy Black man except for my problem with having a bowel movement. This is where the role of being your own self-advocate and the importance of education about the symptoms of colon cancer becomes important. I had the symptoms but was not aware of them, and I did not voice them in a manner to my doctor that would imply this was something serious.

And I was scared. I now know being a part of the decisions being made about your health and managing your health care plan is as much your responsibility as your doctor's. Symptoms that worsen and continue to impact your well-being, such as not having a normal bowel movement every day, straining for what seemed like hours, and mentally challenging your state of mind need to be addressed.

You need to actively participate in plans to care for yourself. Your pride, fear, and being unaware of resources available to help you all impede early screening, which can save your life.

My doctor never talked about the colonoscopy test. It was never in the conversation – when I went to my doctor, he just said to take some stool softeners and some Miralax. He said I needed more fiber in my body. That was about it. I don't think he took it as seriously as it really was, and I wish we both would have.

But because I was really starting to get concerned, I started paying more attention and researching my problems. I talked to different people, and someone I respected told me that Black men need to get their colonoscopy test at 40. That stuck in my head. If I hadn't heard that, I wouldn't be around to write this book.

THE NEXT CHAPTER: ESSL

As soon as I heard more details about the colonoscopy, I didn't say what I was thinking: 'I'm not going to let them put the glove and grease on, go up in there… no man is playing with my butt.' It didn't matter if I wouldn't feel anything under anesthesia. Everything about it was just dead wrong.

Instead, I just told people, "Okay. I'll look into it." But I knew it wasn't going to happen – because I believed it would work out if I just gave it time, and I would be all right. Right? Besides, I wasn't about to consider a colonoscopy paying out of pocket. It could cost anywhere from $1,500 to $4,000 without insurance depending on what needed to be done once they got in there.

Since I was traveling back and forth between Asheville and Charlotte for my businesses, trying to have a bowel movement on the road in public men's rooms is really a joke when your system isn't working the way it's supposed to. Guys would be walking in and out to use the urinals and there I'd be, sitting and waiting, sitting and waiting, wondering who else might like to get in that little stall, too.

We all know it's easiest to relax in your home bathroom, so things were better in Asheville. But in Charlotte and on the road, it wasn't going well. I had cramps and pressure like I needed to go, but no matter how long I waited, it was a whole lot of nothing for all the discomfort.

AVOIDANCE

The colonoscopy test began lurking closer and closer in the back of my mind. With Mama's background as a nurse, a cancer survivor, and a community activist, she had already expressed her opinion on the subject. She worked with a program that was called Project Access to help people without insurance in the healthcare world. She helped educate people on ways they could overcome obstacles to getting the proper medical care.

"There are ways to help pay for the costs for a colonoscopy, such as Project Access," she said. "You don't have insurance and this program can provide the financial assistance you need for a colonoscopy. Your doctor starts the process by writing a referral. The sooner you get it done, the better off you'll be. You'll finally get some answers."

But how often do we listen to our mothers? Only when we find out later that they were right. I had been doing this entrepreneur work, booking parties, shows, and concerts for about 20 years by then. I'm happy that work got me to where I'm at now, but I had never seen the real money part of creating the shows. I kept going in the process and I took my losses like a man —more losses than wins. There is a lot of stress in the life of an entrepreneur.

Because I work for myself, I don't have insurance. My first financial priority is to do right by my kids, and next in line after that is investing back into my businesses. I reluctantly began searching for a way to get insurance that would cover it. Absolutely no insurance companies would pay for a colonoscopy test until I turned 45. It didn't matter if I was having symptoms. Without a doctor's orders, it was not covered.

Well, that was that. I wasn't thrilled with the idea of the test anyway, and for sure, I didn't have the money to pay out thousands of dollars to have it. It seemed to me that the best way forward was to change my diet even more to be a little healthier and try to lower the stress in my life. Neither of those proved to be easy things to do. But I had hope that in time, everything would clear up.

But things weren't getting any better. In fact, they were getting worse. I started seeing blood in my stool. And because it had happened just once in a while a few times before, I figured I must have hemorrhoids again and it would just go away. But deep inside, I think I knew I was heading into something bad. Just like most of us, though, I couldn't accept that at first. I began to will my body to get better. If I just kept up eating healthier foods and cutting down on stress, it would clear up from the changes I was making. I really tried to believe that.

The time came when I decided I should at least check into other ways to cover the cost of the test. I would be turning 40 soon, and someone I trusted warned me that I might have something serious going on. At a different time in my life, I might have waved that off, but not anymore. Imagine what people without insurance have to go through in the face of life-threatening diseases. How will they pay for all of that?

I have been volunteering for years for a nonprofit called My Daddy Taught Me That, a youth development program designed to support young men through advocacy, education, and mentoring. In addition, I have produced hundreds of urban comedy shows in Asheville that brought our community a lot of healing through laughter. The concerts I produced in North Carolina and other states nearby also had provided me with a number of great contacts and friends.

From all these connections and being a community activist myself, and seeing Mama's work with Project Access, I was able to ask for help with getting my colonoscopy test paid for from Project Access, too. In December, I could finally schedule the test.

In January, I was turning 40, and my colonoscopy test was scheduled for the week of my birthday. But come on, this was a BIG birthday, and I was about to turn up! So, I decided to reschedule that one – wouldn't you?

I went ahead and bought the solution they wanted me to drink for the prep, but it sat there on a shelf waiting for me. I avoided looking at it. I didn't want to deal with the what if's, the feelings of fear before and after drinking it, and the uncertainty of it all. I didn't want that feeling even though I needed to do what I had to do.

Then came March 2020. Even though I had the solution right there with me, I didn't take it yet because the facility where I was originally scheduled stopped taking patients due to COVID. So I had to wait in line to schedule the test at the hospital, and that required even more funding because costs are higher at a hospital than at an outpatient facility.

COVID in 2020 was a crazy time for everyone, and especially for everyone working in health care. There wasn't a lot of communication going on. And of course, I dropped the ball because I didn't drink the solution when I was supposed to in time for the first appointment they had for me in February. I was procrastinating because I really didn't want to take the test or drink that stuff, but I knew I had to do it. So they had to try to reschedule me. They were full up in March. Then came a chance for April 17th.

By this time, Mama was nearly beside herself with frustration. "You need to get this test done. You're having trouble moving your bowels. Go see what's going on!"

"All right," I agreed. "Let me get it over with."

Making the decision to finally have a colonoscopy was hard. I didn't really know what to expect, and I had a fear of being violated and humiliated. And I was frustrated that my digestive problems kept getting worse. Even with all the anxiety, anger, frustration and fear, I was tired and I knew I needed answers, but I didn't know what this might all turn into.

Things were really challenging now. I wasn't having a bowel movement for days, and even after having one, I was mentally and emotionally in a downward spiral. I didn't know what would happen before, during, and after the colonoscopy. I felt violated before I even arrived at the hospital, but there was no turning back. The unknown had to be known. But damn, I never expected cancer.

Thinking back on it all, I remember all the ways in which I put off this test trying to be a tough man. A truly tough man takes care of his body first because without a strong, healthy body and mental state, he can't take care of his family and his business. So I have this to say to the men in my community especially:

Don't Wait 'til the Last Minute . . . Go Get Checked!

CHAPTER 3

AWAKENING

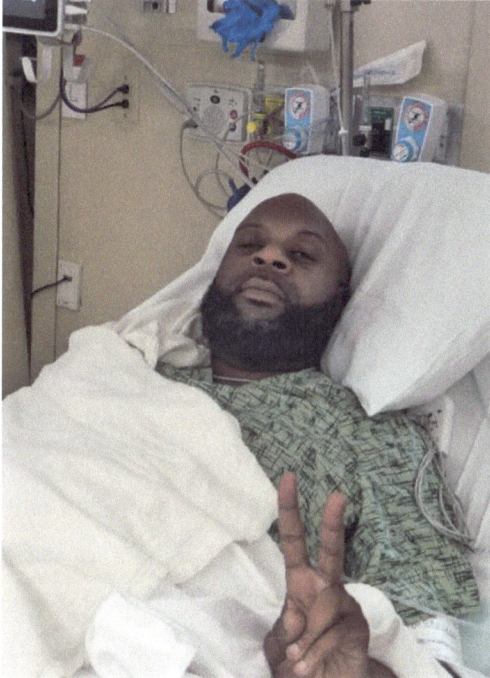

On April 17th, I finally drank the solution. It came in a smaller bottle than I had been expecting. Others had told me about their experiences drinking a big gallon bottle of terrible-tasting stuff. But I got a little bitty bottle. I took the solution and followed all the instructions. I was able to get it down real easy – it was nowhere near as bad as I had been told.

AWAKENING

My dad drove me to the hospital. Sitting next to him in the waiting room, I acted like it was just a minor annoyance. "Well, I'm here, so let me do this little test and get it out of the way."

They called me back and put an IV in my wrist after they made sure I had done the entire protocol correctly. The bed I was on was a wheeled stretcher, and they rolled me into another room.

"Mr. Greene, please get up on this examining table," the nurse asked. As I was transferring to that, she stopped me. "Wait. What do you have on under there?"

"I've got my underwear," I replied confidently. If someone had told me to take that off, I sure hadn't heard it. Maybe I didn't want to.

"Oh no, baby, you gotta take those off," she said and gave me a look. Great. So there I was having to take my underwear off. I wasn't exactly thrilled at this point. "Okay," she continued, "We're starting the anesthetic drip now to put you to sleep for the procedure. Start counting down from 5 to 1 for me, please."

I didn't remember anything after 5, 4, 3 until I started waking up. Through the fog in my head, I heard the nurse saying, "The doctor will be in to see you in a few minutes."

Wow, I thought. That was so easy. I went to sleep like a light going out, and when I woke up, my colonoscopy was done. I didn't feel a thing.

"Now, we need you to pass gas if you can," she encouraged me. "I'll leave you alone for that, but you let me know if it worked."

No problem. It didn't hurt or anything. I want to give all of this information out coming from a Black man because I know how hard it is to share such personal experiences with other men.

I could feel my body slowly coming back to life. Things were starting to be a little more clear. The doctor walked in and asked how I was feeling. He had a very serious expression on his face and paused for a second. "Well, Mr. Greene, I hate to inform you that you've got cancer. You've got colon cancer."

"Damn." That was the first word out of my mouth. The second words were, "Well, what's the next move? I got kids. What do we need to be doing then?"

"I'm going to refer you to my specialist," he said. "We need to get you in for surgery as soon as possible."

My mind was racing at this point. I had played football as a starter in high school and college. I had some injuries back in the day, but I never had any major surgery. While I was getting dressed and heading out from the recovery room, I was in a daze. This was not information you could just shake off. By the time they walked me out to meet Dad, I didn't have to say much about it. He took one look at my face and knew.

"It's cancer," I said when we got to the car. "They want to do surgery."

He took a deep breath. "I love you," he said, shaking his head, and put the car in drive. When we got to my home, I asked him to tell Mama to call me.

She came up and sat at my kitchen table with me. Even as I started to speak, she said, "I know."

The tears rolled down my face. I was numb and afraid at the same time. I told her, "The doctor said I have cancer. I can't take in the full impact of those words. I didn't think I would ever hear that said to me. This never entered my mind."

Mama put her arms around me and held me close. She wiped the tears rolling down my face and kissed me softly so many times. She whispered, "God has you, son, and so do I."

Right after receiving news like that, I didn't really understand it yet, but I was going through it. It's like getting on a train because you have to, but not really knowing where it's going to take you. It took going home and sitting down and being by myself, then breaking the news to the rest of my family. That's when I began to process it a little more. I texted my siblings and close family members about my cancer diagnosis. Putting the words in a text rather than saying them gave me the emotional state of mind I needed to try and let it sink in.

I didn't want to talk to anyone. I knew they loved me, but I could not handle their emotions and my emotions. I asked them for space and time, and they gave me space and time. But they also gave me unconditional support and their time just being with me. Being with me whether in person, a text message, or a phone call. They were at a distance from me but never far away.

My family knew how life can be, and they took it in stride. They accepted that we were all going to have a battle on our hands, and they knew I was going to fight hard for my life.

After my dad's dialysis treatments and kidney transplant a few years before, he was already very familiar with the medical world. Mama's successful battle with ovarian cancer and being a nurse and healthcare advocate prepared her for being my support.

Since I had gone through all those medical challenges with my parents personally, maybe my road ahead looked a little less scary than it might have been for someone else. However, I was much younger than my parents had been, and cancer tends to grow more quickly the younger you are. I found myself thinking about my kids a lot while I waited to talk with the specialist. I felt I needed my kids more than they needed me.

Everyone remarked on how quiet I became. They weren't used to that from me.

After all those months of delays, they got me in for a rush appointment to see the specialist within three days. On April 20th, I sat down with the surgeon.

"Here's what's happening. You have Stage 3 cancer, and once people get to Stage 4, it's usually the end of the game," he told me. "At that point, we would have to remove enough of your colon in surgery that you would have to wear a colostomy bag, possibly forever. If you had waited just a few weeks longer, you might have been at Stage 4."

I already knew what a colostomy bag was. It hooks up under your clothes and collects all your stool because you are no longer having a bowel movement the natural way. To me, this seemed worse than death. We looked at each other in silence for a minute as he gave me time to let it sink in.

"I can't accept this," I told him. "I have too much to live for, and too many people counting on me. What do I have to do to beat this thing?"

He nodded. "Joe, you're 40, you're healthy, you don't smoke cigarettes, and you don't eat red meat." He looked down at my chart and paused as he read it again. "You don't have the triggers or the genetics for what's going on in your body. You're 40; I'm only 44. I'm going to treat you like my brother, and we are going to get this out of you."

"That's cool," I said. "Let's go!"

He got me scheduled for emergency surgery on April 27th, seven days later. That was the longest seven days of my life.

CHAPTER 4

EMERGENCY SURGERY

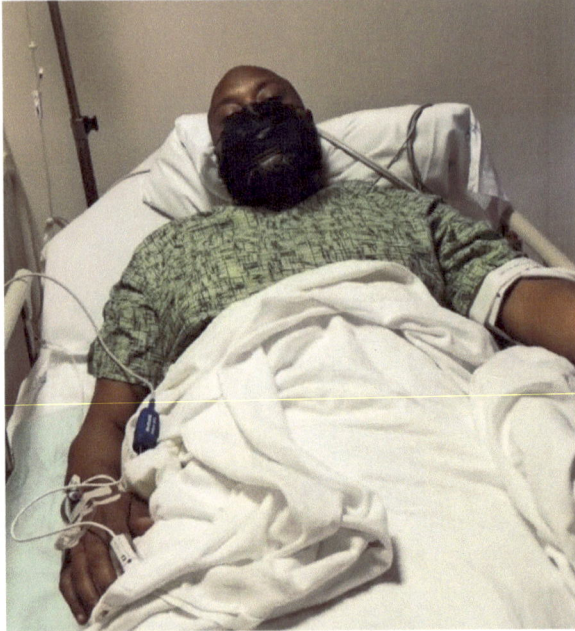

The prep for the surgery was the same as the colonoscopy prep, but they also gave me some extra immune-boosting drinks, because they wanted my body to be strong enough during the procedure. The surgery was scheduled for 9 am on April 27. We had to be there by 8 am, so Mama and I headed out early.

While we were in the waiting room, I was still trying to process everything, so Mama filled out the paperwork for me. This was my first serious surgery. The only other one I had was for my kneecap, which was just a day in, day out surgery. I didn't really know what to expect or what was going to go on. I was just trying to go with the wave. I was glad Mama was there to take care of some things so I could keep myself steady.

"Mr. Greene? We're ready for you," the nurse announced promptly at 9:00.

"Here we go," I said to Mama in a resigned voice, but she saw the worry in my eyes. She squeezed my hand, prayed, and kissed my forehead. In the first room, I had to get out of my clothes, get into the gown, and lay down on the bed. The nurses were very efficient and took good care of me, getting me ready and putting in my IV. It all seemed so routine to them but I still felt like I was in some kind of alternate universe. I just laid there on the bed, taking it all in as much as I could, watching everything they were doing.

From that first room, I announced my surgery to the world through Facebook. I told my whole story. I said I was about to go into surgery, and that I wasn't sharing that right now for anyone's sympathy – I was sharing it with all my followers hoping to inspire the next man to go get his colonoscopy test. "We can feel good on the outside," I told them, "but we don't know what's going on inside our bodies."

While I was making my post, this was all so new and unreal to me, telling everyone I have colon cancer. The whole time I kept spelling it cologne cancer. It was all so hard to grasp and take in. As I was finishing up that post, I shut the phone off because they called my name to go back to surgery.

From there, I had to switch to another bed and they rolled me back into the surgery room. There were a lot of medical instruments and machines in there, a lot of people walking around with masks on, goggles on, surgery gowns. It was cold. I could feel a chill in the air and it seemed to seep down into my lungs and my bones.

Of course I was nervous, but I couldn't let the nerves take over me. I had to be strong. I stopped looking around, made myself stop thinking about stuff, and I was just there. I wasn't really scared, but it was an unsettling feeling. I pulled my mind toward one central thought: I don't accept this cancer. From day one, I've never accepted it, and I still don't accept it. I never will accept it. It has become my frame of mind during this whole process, and it gives me strength.

The anesthesiologist told me that I would be completely asleep during the entire surgery.

My doctor came in, talking to me through his mask. "Joe, we've got a great team here today to get you through this surgery. I'll keep you fully informed about everything we find and everything we were able to do when you wake up, but you are not going to feel a thing. Are you feeling all right?" His eyes were kind and reassuring.

"Yes, sir," I said, looking back up at him steadily. "Thank you." All I could think about in that moment was how fast everything had happened – 10 days ago, I was having a colonoscopy and now here I was having emergency surgery. Remember, this could be you!

"All right, then," he said, nodding over at the anesthesiologist.

Just as in the colonoscopy, I was asked to count backwards from 10. I only remember saying, "10, 9, 8 . . ." Those drugs are something else.

When I first woke up from surgery, I looked around a quiet room with plain white walls. It was still so cold in there. My nose was full of snot and my throat was sore from the tube they had to stick down my throat. I was feeling very foggy from the anesthesia, but they had Mama join me in the recovery room to hear what the doctor had to say.

"Joe, we removed a mass from you about the size of a tennis ball," the doctor told us. He held up his hands to show us how big it was. Mama caught her breath and I just stared at his hands. "We needed to make 7 incisions, and those will heal up just fine."

He went on to explain that there are layers and layers of intestinal walls, and the cancer grows into those areas that can't be seen during surgery. "We did remove one section of your colon that was closest to the tumor we took. But we don't want to take more sections of your colon out because that will affect your quality of life. You will need chemo treatments to kill the rest of the cancer completely."

Mama nodded. I'm sure she knew all along what he was going to say. I kept thinking about pieces of my insides being cut out, and decided to stop focusing on that.

"What are the next steps?" I asked. That's always my question. Got to keep moving on.

"You'll need some time to recover and get your body working again. The nurses will explain what to do, and we'll call you soon to get your first chemo treatment scheduled." He gave us an encouraging look. "You're a strong young man, Joe. We are going to do everything we can to work with you to get you free of cancer."

When the surgery medication wore off, the pain really hit me. I wished many times that the pain medicines they gave me after surgery could be as effective as the anesthesia. They told me while I lay there trapped in that bed that I wouldn't be able to get out of the hospital until I was able to successfully move my bowels. I hadn't had anything resembling a real bowel movement for a long time, and now I was required to pull that off or I'd be stuck in there even longer. Not only that, but they needed to see me get up and walk around on my own, too.

The nurses were good about giving me more pain medicine, but I kept feeling the pain in my stomach where they took the tumor out of me. The wake-up is the real challenge of the surgery, when you're waking up and your body is responding to what just happened, and what will be happening. In my mind, I was trying to imagine that a couple weeks ago, I couldn't make my bowels work at all, and now I was thinking, 'Can I use the bathroom now? Did the surgery really work?'

"C'mon, Joe," the nurse said. "Let's get you walking now." They got me up and moving around right after surgery. I had to walk laps around the floor I was on to avoid getting blood clots, pulling my IV pole with me.

I had to eat whether I felt like it or not, and I had to be able to pass gas, pee, and move my bowels. They watched me like a hawk for all these things. It's a different kind of life with absolutely no privacy!

I had turned my phone off to go into surgery. So, imagine now, I turned my phone back on the next day after the surgery because I was too sore to really deal with it the night before. As soon as the phone powered up, there were all these messages, questions, love – all kinds of stuff.

Mind you, I'm the kind of person who's never been on that side of the track. I'm always the one who motivates, giving the message of encouragement, like, "Let's keep pushing," or "Everything's going to be fine." I was never the one who had to be on the receiving end, to receive the love and sympathy.

I didn't know how to take it. I still don't know how to take it right now, to be honest with you. When people ask me if I'm okay, I appreciate what they're doing, but I don't want to be that sick guy. I don't even move like that.

If they didn't know what was going on with my cancer battle, nobody would ask me those questions anyway. I understand it's coming from a caring place, but people don't understand that it's hard for me to accept it sometimes. So I had to learn how to accept the love.

The best messages were from people saying, "Thank you for opening my eyes. I'm going to get my colonoscopy test done." During that time, I had probably about 10 to 15 men saying they were going to go get their colonoscopy test done after seeing my post.

From that day on, I thought, well, you know, basically the Lord gave me this challenge. And that was the beginning of an idea that later turned into ESSL, Early Screening Saves Lives.

I was scheduled to be in the hospital 7 days, but I was back in my house in 3 days. I did everything in my power to keep pushing myself. I didn't want to sit around in the hospital for 7 days dwelling on this – I wanted to get back to living.

THE NEXT CHAPTER: ESSL

When I got back home, it took some days to feel normal. Using the bathroom was unpredictable and it was hard not to make everything be about that. I still needed rest and I still needed to heal. I was way more comfortable at home, of course, and I was so happy to be there.

I took a couple weeks off of work, but I never really stopped working; I made things happen for my businesses from my bed.

Even though they took a mass out, they only took what they could see, so the next challenge was getting rid of the rest of the cancer. Can you imagine walking around in your life knowing that there is cancer hiding and growing inside hidden layers of walls in your intestines?

I'm telling you, it's a surreal experience and one that I wouldn't wish on anyone, ever.

I was blessed not to have a full re-section, but since they did take a section of my colon out and sewed the rest of it together, my colon isn't as long as everyone else's anymore. I can't hold as much as the next person anymore.

The cramps are harder now with less colon to do the job. How I break food down is different now. Everything is different.

EMERGENCY SURGERY

I was already scheduled for chemo to begin only 6 weeks after the surgery. Now it was time for my body to enter a major battle to kill off all the cancer they couldn't remove in the surgery.

Once again, I was about to be drawn into a brand-new experience. Even though I had seen Mama's experience with chemo firsthand, this was all new to me.

CHAPTER 5

CHEMO

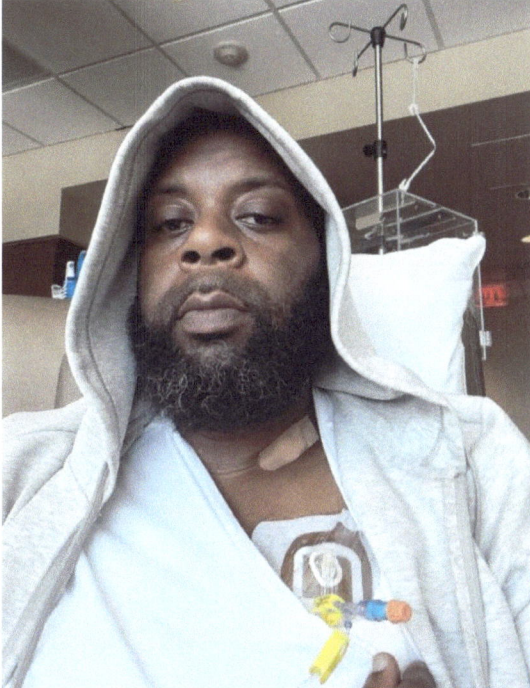

Everyone talks about the side effects of chemo – losing your hair, nausea, weakness, a bad taste in your mouth, and other issues. I had my side effects too, but I learned that I can't really complain about that too much. I've seen how badly chemo affected other people out there. I've seen some people go through some real hardships from this treatment. I was thankful that I was able to face it in the way I faced it, at least for the first round.

CHEMO

A round of chemo is 12 treatments, held every other week for 24 weeks, so that's 6 months of your life invaded by chemicals designed to kill cells. I had my first chemo session about a month and a half after the surgery. I started out with treatments every other Monday morning. I always asked for early sessions, because I wanted to get It out of the way and get back to my day.

Before the sessions started, they had to put a port in my chest. They told me it was a minor procedure, but I really hate needles plus I don't like the idea of someone putting a hole in my chest very much. Thankfully, I didn't have to drink any prep solutions to get the port put in. The port is a little box they embed in your chest. It's a line with a needle that goes into your vein.

They cut me at the top where the vein is, then they put a box shaped like a strip down in there near the top of my chest. They don't put you to sleep when they do your port, but they did put a sheet up so I didn't have to watch. I was glad about that. I remember them numbing my skin and cutting me, and then they said it was done and closed it up. Then that was it.

Even when they put the port in, I didn't really know what a port was. The box pokes out a little bit – even though it's under my skin, I can feel it. It took me a long time to get used to it. They put a Band-Aid over it and told me to take the Band-Aid off later and let the wound heal. But it took me a very long time to take the Band-Aids off there because I just didn't want to look at it. It took me some months!

Another thing about the port: You can't lift weights and use resistance machines – you can only have a certain amount of weight or resistance. You don't want the port to slip or get messed up.

I kept putting a new Band-Aid on because I didn't like that hole being there. It kept me humble since it was nothing I'd been through before, and it was all happening so fast. Something new comes along and you can fight it all you want, but it's still happening. I really avoided getting it wet or touching it because I didn't want it to get infected. I had two cuts on my body. I didn't want to see them and kept them covered.

"Joe, you have to keep those Band-Aids off!" Mama insisted. "Those cuts have to heal up."

I finally started looking at it and it wasn't as bad as I thought it would be. It was still visible. I can just put my hand on my chest now and I feel it. I don't feel it when I'm just moving around, but when I put my hand on my chest, I can feel it there. I don't have to cover it up while taking a shower, because it's underneath my skin.

Mama had a port during her chemo days, but I never understood what it was until they started taking my blood tests from my port.

CHEMO

They don't have to try to find a vein in my arms or hands anymore – they just easily access it through the port in my chest.

After signing in at 8 am for my first chemo session, they took my blood pressure and temperature. If those weren't within normal range, I'd have to come back another time, but mine were okay. They walked me back to the chemo area and told me they were going to access my port.

When they access your port, they have to hit it at a certain spot, because if they poke it at the wrong spot, it hurts like hell. I had someone put the needle in wrong and they tried to force it, and it was a painful experience. The right spot is in the middle of the port, and the nurse is trained to get the correct stick the first time. My skin just grows back over the hole they poke every time, like when they take blood from your vein in your arm.

When they first access your port for each session, they take your blood and send it to the lab. That will tell if your blood levels are at the right range to have the treatments. It's about a 20-minute wait. If your white and red blood cell counts aren't right, your body won't process the chemo like it should. So I waited for my results to come back and see if I could take the treatment that day. I almost hoped they weren't in range, but I also just wanted to get this whole thing over with.

"Well, Joe, your labs look just fine," the nurse told me. "Let's get you started. I'm going to use this needle to inject a saline solution through your port to flush it out so all the medicines can get into your bloodstream successfully."

I held up my hand when I saw the size of the needle she was starting to point at my chest. "I'm sorry, but I have a thing about needles," I told her.

She paused and then smiled at me. "Then you'll just have to look away. This is a very important part of the procedure." I looked away.

The saline going into the port sent this taste into my mouth and nose that I instantly hated. The smell of the alcohol they used for sanitizing drove me crazy, too. I could never get used to these tastes and smells all through my experience with chemo. When I know that I have to get my port flushed, I turn my head every time. I don't have tattoos, and I don't do needles.

They started the medicines dripping down into my IV through my port. The first medicine was for nausea so I wouldn't throw up, so my body could accept all the medicine they were about to put inside me. After that came some pain medicine. Then, they started the chemo. It's a process that takes 4 or 5-hours. You can't feel it when you're getting the chemo treatment, but your smells and taste are different. Weird and unnatural.

CHEMO

The chemo treatment itself wasn't as hard as the process after the treatment. When it was time for me to leave, they gave me a pouch that was attached to my port. This really drove me crazy. The pouch had a medicine ball in it, like the size of a grenade, in a fanny pack.

The grenade was hooked to my port as an attachment, with a bunch of tape around it to keep it still in the port. So all these different medicines just kept on coming through that thing into my bloodstream.

The nurse explained how it worked. "Okay now, you will keep this pouch right here like this for the next 72 hours. This will keep the medicine going to help kill the cancer. You cannot take a shower, and you have to make sure you don't dislodge it from your port while you are resting or sleeping. Prop yourself up in bed so you can't roll over on it."

I stared down at that pouch like I wanted to rip it off my body and throw it across a football field. I had to keep this grenade attachment hanging from my port and take it home and wear it for 72 hours? That's leaving chemo, after 4 to 5 hours, and then going home for 72 more hours of more medicine going into my body. But I held my peace.

"Wednesday will be your Detachment Day. You'll come back here and we'll take this out of your port. After that, you can shower and go about your life as usual." She smiled encouragingly at me.

"Okay. Thank you," I said. I was beginning to have doubts that this was going to be a manageable experience. As the hours ticked on, it felt like I was being slowly poisoned. This really affected my state of mind. I tried to think about positive things but it became harder and harder. It wasn't easy to do regular things or hang out with friends and family acting like everything was just fine.

Sometimes I felt anxious and on edge, like I was in serious danger. Other times, I was just exhausted and mentally depressed.

For the next two days, I didn't take a shower and I couldn't get any decent sleep because that big, uncomfortable medicine ball was there hanging off of me with the pouch stuck around my waist. And there was all that medicine still pumping through my body. The metallic taste that started during the chemo treatment on Monday felt like it was traveling all through my body now, into my pores.

When I went back to get the pouch detached, it had gone from a full, grenade-sized ball to a flattened ball. There had to be no medicine left in it when I went back. When they detached me, I was free to go about my day. But it wasn't really freedom because my body now had to process this huge invasion of medicine. It made me sleepier than usual and having to pee so much more often because of all the fluids.

They told me to drink plenty of water to flush it all out, and the volume of pee rose to a whole different kind of level. My pee was a different color, too. Everything about it just felt wrong.

I was on blood pressure pills from before the cancer diagnosis, and those are like a water pill. It's harder to have a normal bowel movement after all that medicine, too. Although some of the medicines cause diarrhea, some of them will stop up the intestines. I had already suffered from being stopped up way too long, so when the diarrhea hit, I was actually relieved just to be going. But it drained me so much that I became too weak and sometimes got the shakes because I was so dehydrated.

Everything I ate or drank was going right through me, so I finally had to take the anti-diarrhea pill to stop myself up. To tell you the truth, it was one of the best days of my life when I did finally take that pill. It was so good to clear that up.

After that first session, I could feel my adrenalin pumping hard as soon as I got out of the car to go in for a treatment. I'd put my mask on and walk into the building to check in. While I sat there waiting for the nurse to call me and check my weight and my blood pressure, I knew my blood pressure was continuing to rise. My anxiety was building up just being inside this place again.

Every time I got my blood pressure taken, it was high. It didn't matter if I took my blood pressure pills, it was very high. Every time I was in that place, no matter how much I tried to relax, it was the same story. Each time I went, I could be put in a different section.

Sometimes I had somebody next to me on both sides, but they gave us our own space with a curtain around and a wall behind. So it was like being in an open space but you can't see the other people. You can just hear them.

"Would you like a warm blanket?" the nurses would ask. It was always cold in there, I guess to keep the germs down, but it was really cold. I always asked for two blankets. I was starting to have some more side effects as the treatments wore on.

I was losing weight, which made me get cold more quickly, but a big problem was neuropathy. My hands and feet were always cold and numb all day. It takes quite a while to get used to it. I can't take my shoes off and walk on the floor with just my socks on – it hurts. My feet are still numb to this day.

They hooked me up to a machine that pumped the medicines into the port in my chest through a needle, so I needed to stay put during the session. I had an IV pole on rollers, so luckily I could walk to the bathroom with it when I needed to.

They gave me a TV remote, and I had my phone while I sat there. Some people take a nap because the medicines don't hurt while they are being pumped into your body. You just have to keep getting up to go pee, because all of that fluid going into your body.

They also tell you to drink water so you can try to flush your body during the session and afterward. They also want you to get up and walk afterward so it moves the medicine through your body more efficiently.

Chemo causes exhaustion. It's going to lay you down no matter how strong you think you are. And it's very common to feel isolated, like you're living in a different nightmare dimension that no one with a "regular" life could understand.

Sometimes people feel they have to shield their families from being a part of the treatment, but having a support person there with you can be a big help.

Some people really need someone there but may not realize they have that option. I had to find a way to fight that feeling of isolation because I could feel it trying to drown my spirit, so my family made sure someone was there with me at each chemo session.

Besides all that, the taste in your mouth is not a taste I would wish on anybody. I could brush my tongue a thousand times, but that taste would never go away. I didn't get much nausea because I smoked weed. They asked me to see if I could switch to the gummies, but they weren't for me. So, I'm back to smoking it. It has helped me a lot through this whole process to this day.

Another thing that has helped me tremendously was switching to a plant-based diet. Right after I was diagnosed with colon cancer, I made a phone call to a childhood friend of mine, Damion Bailey. He had gone through colon cancer about 3 years before that, and he shared his journey with us through Facebook. He didn't smoke, drink, or have any bad habits, and he ended up having colon cancer. He is now cancer-free and maintaining a healthy life and diet.

I called him and told him what was going on. He sent me a list of movies to watch, and I included those in the More Information section at the back of this book. I also listed his book recommendations in the Resources section. He said I should look into a different way of eating that had helped him beat cancer.

He listed different stuff to start adding to my diet like alkaline water, turmeric, ginger, vitamin D3, ginseng, liquid chlorophyll, sea moss, black seed oil, dandelion root, and bladderwrack in addition to switching over to all fruits and vegetables and plant-based food.

He stressed the importance of detoxing every week with a colon cleanse if I remained constipated. It worked for him and I have tried it, too, but everyone should decide what's best for their body.

I started watching the movies, like "What the Health." I learned about how they produce the fish, the chicken, the meat – all the bacteria and antibiotics that goes into the food. What we eat is literally taking us out. When I had my surgery, they took a huge mass out of me. I told myself that if they took all of that out of me, I'm not going to put it back in me.

From that day on, I became plant-based. I don't eat fish, chicken, red meat, none of that. Yellow cheese isn't good for you because of the oils they use during processing and the antibiotics they pump into the cows – it's about as bad as meat. That actually helped me out, because I asked for a challenge and eating this way has been a challenge from all different angles.

Now I'm eating fruits and vegetables, something I haven't done in years. I had to go back to eating eggs because I wasn't getting enough protein in my body. If your blood cell counts are not right when you go to chemo, they won't treat you. So, I had to go back to eating eggs to get enough protein.

"Joe, I want you to start eating fish at least twice a week," one of the nurses told me. "Your protein is still on the low side."

I shook my head. I was determined not to let that sickness back into my body. "No, I'm not doing that," I said. "What are the other options?"

"Well, you could try some protein shakes," she said. I could tell she didn't think that would do the trick, but it did. And it wasn't easy for me, either. Ever since I went into chemo treatment, I found I couldn't drink or eat anything cold. Ice is my enemy, period. My fingertips turn different colors, and I can't put my hands in the freezer or the refrigerator. If I touch something cold, my fingertips send a shockwave through my body. Neuropathy really affects your quality of life.

These are just some of the things that can happen to people during chemo. If I drink something cold, it feels like swords going down my throat, so all my drinks need to be room temperature.

The whole experience has been an education for me, too. I understand other people's problems and sensitivities much better now. Having cancer has opened my eyes and also the eyes of a lot of other people around me.

Another benefit to plant-based eating was that I could use the restroom now! People don't know how deep that is to you, because it's a norm to everybody. If you're not able to really pass your stool because your body isn't able to break down your food, you can be on the toilet for hours and then get up and there's nothing there. Now, I take the good with the bad. I know it sounds crazy to be so focused on what happens in the bathroom, but there's a lot going on behind the scenes in everyone's life.

Plant-based eating has been a real blessing and has opened my eyes to what the typical American diet really does. I feel good now, and I look good. I can think more clearly, focus better, and I can move my body better since I switched my diet over. It's been a dope little venture. My friends and family have definitely been helpful, riding along with me on my eating journey. They've taken the steps to cut some of the unhealthy stuff out of their diet.

I don't eat fish or chicken or red meat, just vegetables, grains, and fruits, and adding in eggs and protein powder for protein. I miss chicken – chicken was my favorite thing! I liked hot dogs. To switch over and not eat that stuff has been a challenge, but it's been a lifestyle change. It made me think different, it made my skin look different and made me feel different.

Just because they say some things are healthy for you doesn't mean it's healthy for you. I learned that a lot of soy and plant-based sausages and hamburgers, like Impossible Burgers, are not so good for you. The vegan meat substitutes have a taste that just isn't for me. Sometimes I can get by on different things, but I'm not a big fan of the alternative sausages and stuff like that. I really just stick to the veggie parts of stuff.

I got so many different suggestions about what to do from people. I had to sort through all that because everything isn't going to work for everybody. It might work for them, but it might not work for me. I took some of the information and rolled with it, but it had to be right for me.

Portions are different on the plant-based diet. I definitely don't eat like I used to. I'm down 75 lbs. I'm just eating the "sides" of what most people call a meal. Of course, I want my stuff to taste good, too.

"What can I cook for you?" my friends will often ask, because they aren't sure what to offer when they invite me over.

"Just cook it the same as you'd cook a regular meal, but take the meat out of it for me," I tell them. I want the flavor and the seasoning; I want all that. It's hard enough to eat how I'm eating, so I might as well have it seasoned well and tasty.

My kids eat with me, so they rock with me, but not all the time. Sometimes I have to slide the healthy stuff in on them. I don't try to make them change over to plant-based – they know they can choose what they want to eat, and I don't force it on them.

CHEMO

Since I went plant-based and learned to get more protein in my body, my white and red blood cell counts were always good enough to have my chemo treatments.

Keeping up with exercising while doing chemo is another challenge. Getting my body moving and the blood flowing is very important to healing and fighting cancer, but I had to balance it out during chemo. Since my treatments were every other week, on chemo weeks, I was too weak to do my usual 30-minute walk.

I could maybe go for a slow, short walk but I couldn't really push it. My strong week was the week after the session week, and then I would be out there – cold, rain, sleet, didn't matter, I was out there getting my heart rate up no matter how numb my feet were or how uncomfortable it might be.

CHAPTER 6

ADJUSTMENTS

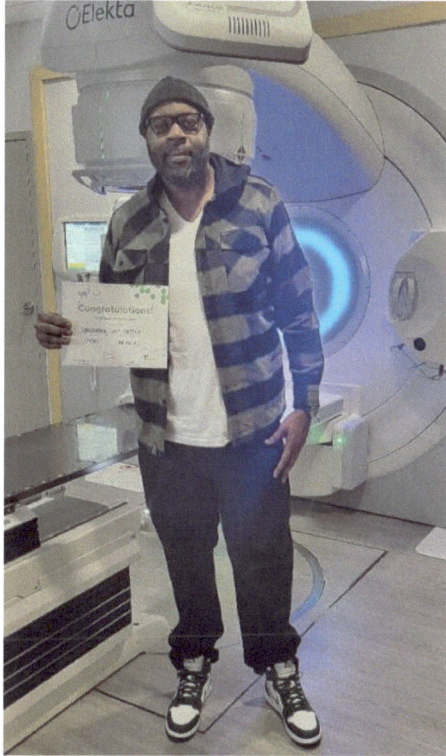

I had completed one round of chemo treatment followed by a round of radiation, which was easier on me than the chemo was. But it was still grueling in its own way — 8 weeks of going in every day, 5 days a week, to get zapped in a big machine. I honestly didn't know how I made it through all that, and I was so ready to ring that bell. That's a ritual they have when you finish a round of treatment. I thought I was done with treatments and could get on with my life now.

But when you finish a whole round of treatments, you get about four weeks off to recuperate, heal, and let the swelling go down from the internal radiation spots. Then they give you a bunch of tests, including a CT and an MRI.

"Joe, your CT scan shows that the cancer is coming back aggressively," my oncologist told me in his office. "It actually grew back in the same spot where we took the original cancer out, so it's still there where we couldn't get it from the intestinal wall during surgery. I've never seen it do that before in anybody."

Wow. Getting that kind of information, I didn't really know what to think, but I didn't want to give in to doom and gloom. The doctor was upbeat about it, though.

"We are going to try chemo again and see what happens," he told me. "With this second round, the doses will be stronger. We need to knock this out before it gets established again in your colon."

Okay, I had been in competitive situations before, and I wanted to fight back. But going through this same routine again for six weeks, knowing that it would be even more difficult to handle, was starting to mess with my mental health. The smells and tastes and the feeling of being poisoned triggered me. I have high blood pressure as it is. Going into chemo messed with my blood pressure.

THE NEXT CHAPTER: ESSL

I've always been very aware of smells, both good and bad. Everything was stronger this time. The odor of the treatment center, just walking in the door, immediately took me to a different place. It's like the PTSD that soldiers have to go through, not being able to control my reactions. Every time I entered the building now to get a chemo treatment, my blood pressure would skyrocket. As soon as a I put that mask on at the entrance, I would get serious anxiety.

I didn't have any anxiety before this cancer journey, but now I was dealing with a powerful urge to run right back out that door. I had to push it down, like a soldier running into a battle. I didn't want to be there, but I had to be there.

It became obvious to my doctors as my mental health spiraled down more and more that this second round of chemo was killing my spirit. It really was a nightmare experience, with the anxiety growing worse and worse. I started losing my hair everywhere on my body.

It really hit me when I watched my beard coming out in clumps, and I would look at myself in the mirror and feel waves of sadness. I never thought losing my hair would be so hard to accept, but it was very visual proof that I was losing control of the battle.

I told everyone on Facebook that I was thankful for my doctors listening to me, because they made an adjustment for me.

ADJUSTMENTS

They looked over my charts and told me, "Well, the radiation we did the first time really hit those spots we were focusing on, so we should try to do it again with the spots that just came up. So it won't be as heavy as the chemo you're going through and not as heavy as the first radiation you went through."

I was beyond thankful and felt blessed. Don't hold back how you really feel when you talk with your doctor. You never know how much they could help you if you just open up.

I did six weeks in radiation therapy, and that's five days a week, so a total of 30 treatments. I was getting my treatments first thing in the morning, getting the kids on the bus, and then going on my way to treatment. I always had breakfast beforehand. Then I would show up at the treatment center for 5 days a week at 8 in the morning, get checked in, and go into a room where the radiation was so strong that my cellphone wouldn't work.

I was in there and out of there in 20 minutes, versus 5 hours sitting there in chemo. With radiation, they don't touch your body, but you feel the soreness and the effects of it quicker than with the chemo. For me, I would rather deal with the soreness than sit through all that time in each chemo session, dealing with the needle in the port in my chest, and sitting there all day.

It's not easy, but I would choose 20-minute radiation sessions over the chemo, though radiation treatments come with their own set of challenges.

The radiation machine is a big gray machine with a hard table. They put a sheet over the table and I would lay on the sheet on my back. Then they marked my stomach with temporary tattoos and stickers so they would get the right spot each time they turned on the radiation. The machine rotated around me.

It wasn't loud, but I could hear it floating around me and I could see the beams. Even during radiation, I kept my eyes closed. Sometimes I could relax, and even doze off for a second. I would keep my mind busy thinking of the projects I had going on – anything positive.

I could feel the rays from the radiation, especially when it was rotating around my body, but it didn't affect me until I left. I would lay there thinking, 'I'm in this machine and it's not touching me, but it's shooting me with rays.' I might not have felt it directly, but I could feel how strong it was. When my body settled down from the treatment, I had to get some rest. The soreness would get worse afterward. They told me to take Tylenol to help the pain.

When I took a shower later, I would look down and see those stickers. It was a constant reminder of the new reality of my life. I don't like needles and I don't like being in machines, but that has been my life since I was diagnosed.

When I was doing radiation treatments, I was still doing chemo, but they were chemo pills. They are the size of horse pills, and I had to take 8 a day, on top of all of the other medicine I was already taking. I had to make sure to eat before taking those pills because they are too strong on an empty stomach. I took 4 in the morning and 4 at night.

They were powerful pills, and the feeling of being poisoned returned. They made my mouth bleed and made my gums real sore. The nurses would always ask if I had sores in my mouth from the chemo pills. The pills built acid in my stomach, too, and they shifted my bowel movements. They can cause diarrhea or stop people up. I had both.

Even though it was a relief to be spared the grueling chemo treatments, I obviously wasn't thrilled with radiation.

"How's the new treatment going?" a friend asked after I switched over from chemo.

"I mean, it's easier than the chemo," I told him. "But damn, I'm in this machine five days a week for six weeks, then I have to take eight pills a day on top of my other pills. These are BIG pills and they give you diarrhea out of this world. My skin is peeling and burnt in spots."

My friend shook his head in sympathy. He looked scared, and I didn't blame him. "Man, that's terrible," he said.

"Yeah. All these treatments do different things to your body. I don't like radiation neither."

I finished my radiation, but I will have to go back again. My fight with cancer is never going to be over. I have 4 weeks off, then I get back into the MRI and have a CT scan to see if the radiation worked this time or didn't work – then we go from there. If the radiation didn't work, I already explained to my doctors that I don't want to go back through chemo again. I don't think I can really do it. I'm strong in a lot of ways, but I don't want to go through that again. I'm not sure what that will mean in terms of next steps if we get bad news.

CHAPTER 7

ACCEPTANCE

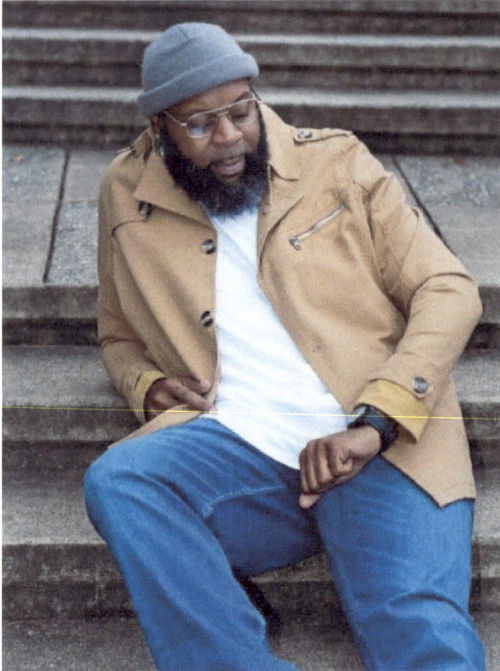

During the Covid time, I was praying for a challenge in life. After all my experiences as a promoter in the entertainment industry, I had learned how to get the word out, establish a fan base, and spread information to the general public. I realized these experiences were like a platform for me to use to raise awareness about what's going on behind the scenes of this colonoscopy issue.

This experience woke my family up, woke the people around me up. It woke me up. People aren't talking about Black health. Even with me fighting like I am now to this day. I'm not saying I'm going to change the world overnight. Black health is just not a conversation that people are having, and when they do have it, it's too late. It's hard to really come back when it's too late. When I say it's too late, I mean you get the news that you're at Stage 4 cancer.

It's hard to come back from stage 4 cancer. It's hard to come back from Stage 3 cancer and I'm Stage 3. I'm not saying that I'm back, but I'm fighting. We wait until the last end to figure it out and only go get the colonoscopy when things are really bad.

But we could have gotten the test done when it was just polyps in the colon, when the cancer hadn't even formed yet. Polyps are signs of cancer. You can probably catch it so much earlier when you're in the polyps stage and be able to fight it easier. When you're in the fourth quarter, it's much more rough.

Here are the symptoms of colon cancer according to the CDC, American Cancer Society, and Mayo Clinic (see Resources section):

- Changes in bowel movements
- Abnormal stools
- Blood in or on your bowel movement (tar-like stool indicates bleeding from higher in the colon while bright red blood is an indicator of bleeding in the lower colon)

- Abdominal discomfort that won't go away: Stomach pain, stomachaches, pelvic pain, stomach cramps, gas and belching
- Nausea and vomiting
- Loss of appetite
- Unexplained weight loss
- Unexplained fatigue or feeling tired
- Anemia
- Shortness of Breath
- Diarrhea, constipation, or feeling that the bowel does not empty all the way.

My mission now is to get this message out to the world and expand public pressure on the policymakers to get 40 years old as the standard age for a first colonoscopy. That's a start. If I would have waited until I was 45, I wouldn't have made it at Stage 3 because at Stage 4, you're facing the end of the game.

And honestly, the age for colonoscopy should be even earlier than 40 because of the food we're getting. The food that goes into our bodies is making us sick. Black men are the number one segment of the population dying from colon cancer, and it's on the rise.

So now, my kids need to get their colonoscopy tests at age 30, since I was diagnosed at 40. We have to get these numbers down, especially for the uninsured people.

Even if you go to the doctor now and say you want a colonoscopy test and you're under 45, they can't order the test unless you have blood in your stool or you're really suffering. They are required by the insurance companies to try everything else first, and while all that is going on, the cancer is quietly growing inside you.

I'm trying to stop people from going through all of this stuff. I still have a port in my chest for chemo. That's what you have to go through, and once cancer gets its hooks into you, the port stays just so it's there for the next time around.

I'll be fighting this cancer all my life, from what I understand. I decided to write a book, to go completely public about everything on Facebook, to give interviews and talks anywhere and anytime I can, just to give people the back end, the raw, uncut story of what's really going on.

I say it over and over: "This conversation has to happen coming from a Black man, and this ain't nothing I heard, this is where I live at." I'm in this fight, and I want to go nationwide talking about this colonoscopy test. Early Screening Saves Lives! ESSL. I really want to put it out there, and I'm hoping I can save the next person. This is what I'm meant to do.

My goal with ESSL is to get the word out about it so people, especially in my community, understand that early detection really saves lives. I never heard a Black man talking about this stuff, ever. It doesn't matter if it is on TV or the Internet. Especially in my world that I've been a part of, I've never heard a Black man talking about it.

I want to go to the colleges and speak. I'm a businessman in the entertainment field, and I want to bring the message. I want to go to the medical facilities, churches, libraries, organizations – you name it. My mission is to spread the word of ESSL. I want to change the numbers. If we at least get it down to being covered at 40, we are making some progress.

Writing this book has helped me create a platform for speaking engagements. I want to answer questions, and I don't want to leave any questions unanswered. We have to educate the people and create a public outcry to bring pressure on lawmakers to change the guidelines for colonoscopy testing. Starting ESSL is a strong first step, but it is just the beginning of the fight to create a consistent, powerful legislative advocacy and lobby for this critical change and save lives.

I appreciate this opportunity to tell my story. A lot of people don't open up about their stories. I get a lot of inboxes from people who don't want to share their stories out loud. I tell them I get it – I know you all are not me, and we aren't going about it the same way, but this is my way.

THE NEXT CHAPTER: ESSL

I want to give you all an honest behind-the-scenes look at this stuff. I want to get the real truth out so you know what you're fighting against and you can be prepared and live your best life.

As I wrote to my Facebook followers: "I got a lot to do here in life still & I'm gonna keep pushing, SCREAMING E.S.S.L.! EARLY SCREENING SAVES LIVES! Now my fight is not over but I'm going to keep smiling, keep living, and keep educating my people through my journey of colon cancer."

The BLACK Spokesman for Colonoscopy Testing at the Age of 40 AMBASSADOR Joe Greene

This Ain't Nothing I Heard.... THIS IS WHAT I'M LIVING 💯 💯 💯

#FCancer   #Salute

FROM MY HEALTHCARE TEAM
AND SUPPORT NETWORK

From Martin Palmeri, MD, MBA
Oncologist

People ask me, "Why would you ever want to be a cancer doctor?" and the answer is simple: I hate cancer. My mother and father both faced cancer diagnoses. I know the fear of having a loved one's cancer return, the hope that a treatment is working, the joy when the CAT scan is looking better, and devastation when the cancer comes back. Knowing how cancer has touched my life, I want to do everything I can to support my patients, offer them the best and most cutting-edge treatments and give them the strength to get through their personal journey.

Although many cancers are unavoidable, some are very preventable. Colorectal cancer is a leading cause of cancer related deaths in the United States and is also one of the most preventable. "Pre-cancers" or colon polyps are easily treatable, and screening can essentially prevent people from getting colon cancer. Yet, 40% of Americans do not go for colon cancer screening.

African American males have some of the highest risks for developing and dying from colon cancer and unfortunately, have some of the lowest screening rates. I have asked several of my African American patients over the years why they don't go for screening, and many do not trust having a nerdy white guy insert a three-foot tube in their rectum. This unfortunately is the result of a history of embedded racism and social health inequities.

I personally do not enjoy doing rectal exams; that is not what inspired me to become a doctor. At the end of the day, if I do NOT do the exam, I could miss a cancer. If I miss diagnosing a cancer, I miss saving that patient and their family all the pain, fear, and suffering my family and I experienced. No matter how embarrassing and uncomfortable it is, preventing cancer is worth it.

At the end of the day, getting screened for colon cancer is better than having to go for surgery to have part of your bowel removed. Screening is better than having a bag to collect feces permanently attached to your abdomen. Screening is better than the fear, suffering and pain caused by having a terminal cancer. Early screening saves lives and at the end of the day we all need to swallow our pride, get screened, and hopefully, never get colon cancer.

From Joseph R. Kelley, MD, PhD
Radiation Oncologist

Early detection is the most important part of cancer treatment. When tumors are small, treatment can be extremely effective and the side effects from therapy are often mild. Unfortunately, if cancer is diagnosed at an advanced stage, treatment is much more difficult for patients and it is more likely that tumors will recur. The key to a good outcome is finding the cancer early.

Going to the doctor for cancer screening is inconvenient and it can be embarrassing to talk with your providers about symptoms, but it is one of the most important things that you can do to protect your health. Mammograms save lives. Pap smears save lives. Colonoscopies save lives.

Getting your PSA checked and asking your provider to examine your prostate is the difference between a good outcome and the horror stories that everyone has heard about cancer treatment. The best thing a patient can do to prevent a problem from cancer is to ask your healthcare provider if you need any cancer screening at the end of each visit.

From Quinton V. Cancel, MD

Oncologic Surgeon

I have had the privilege to work with Joe during his cancer journey on a couple of outreach projects and have witnessed him handle the ups and downs in his fight with great optimism and courage. His relentless spirit and willingness to spread the word on early detection, no matter how sick he feels from treatments or how challenging the prognosis, is inspiring.

He is a living testament to the power of positive thinking and the impact it has on this battle. Joe is on a divine mission to help others, and his efforts have made and will continue to make a difference in the fight for victory over this disease.

From (Mama) Yvette Jives, CEO/LPN/MSW
Cancer Survivor, Author, Activist, and Founder of HERS LLC

I was diagnosed with Stage 2 Ovarian cancer in 2012. My symptoms persisted for months with pelvic pressure, low back pain, urinary frequency and urgency. I followed up with my primary care provider three times within a four-week span and was told each time I had a urinary tract infection, or it may be due to my getting older. I was placed on the same antibiotics twice with no improvement. In fact, my symptoms worsened, and the pain increased.

I advocated for myself and contacted my GYN doctor. I am a nurse, so I questioned my doctor's methods of diagnosing me and his prescribed treatments. Upon hearing my concerns and symptoms, my GYN provider scheduled me for an appointment the same day.

My pelvic exam was unbearable due to a cream my primary care doctor prescribed, but also my exam was determined to have abnormal findings according to my GYN doctor. She ordered a vaginal ultrasound and a CA125 test. My doctor had completed a partial hysterectomy on me in 1997 and she voiced to me that her findings were concerning. At the time I had no idea what a CA125 test was and she never informed me. The lab informed me it was an antigen for a tumor marker for cancer. The CA125 test was repeated twice because the results doubled, and an MRI was scheduled.

In November 2012, I was diagnosed with malignant ovarian cancer and scheduled for surgery in December 2012. I underwent 6 months of chemotherapy every other Monday and finished my last treatment May 13, 2013. I remember the day well because I graduated with my MSW on May 11, 2013. From 2013 until 2022, I went from monthly visits with my GYN/cancer specialist to every 6 months until last year when I was scheduled my first yearly visit.

Listening to your body and being your own advocate is important. But also being informed of and being a part of the decisions made related to your care is so essential, as well as continued follow-through on your plan of care with doctor appointments, discussing screening options, and knowing your risk due to family histories, and genetic testing. It is critical that you have an active voice in being informed of any test ordered and knowing the reasons for tests.

Ovarian cancer is known as a silent killer because it is symptom-driven. There is not a test to diagnose ovarian cancer and it is not diagnosed through a Pap test. Ovarian cancer has the highest mortality percentages for women of color and for being diagnosed in Stage 3 or 4. Interestingly, Caucasian women have the highest percentage of being diagnosed with ovarian cancer but the lowest mortality percentage.

I created HERS LLC as a result of my diagnosis and the reality of this cancer ranking 5th in cancer deaths for women of color. Ovarian cancer's lack of visibility and awareness throughout our communities has impacted women of color generation after generation.

Please visit my website (www.hersnc.org) for information on services provided by HERS LLC and to obtain a copy of my book, *Windowed Revelation of Ovarian Cancer.*

From Trina Gragg-Jackson

Cancer Survivor, Author, and Friend,
Owner of Asheville Pro Lash and Salon

To live is to have been given a gift of fresh air, light, peace, joy, and happiness, but most of all health.

My name is Trina Gragg-Jackson, I am a two-time Breast Cancer Survivor! Winning this case that was set forth upon me makes me feel like the welterweight champion of the world! My gift to this world are my three fabulous children and two beautiful granddaughters. I have been in education for more than 30 years. I have taught over 1800 students in my program area, and at some point in time have had the opportunity to be in the building with over 36,000 students in my 30-year tenure as a North Carolina Educator.

With that being said, I personally have seen a lot and learned a lot. To date I own and operate Asheville Pro Lash and Salon, a 3500 sq. ft. salon and spa. I am the author of *From School to Work for Entrepreneurs in the Beauty Industry*, and a workbook that will help aspiring entrepreneurs through the process. I am the creator of Je La Vois clothing and accessories, Fluff by Trina Clothing for plus-size women, and the owner of The Beauty Coach, a consulting firm for entrepreneurs in the beauty industry.

With all that I do, and all that I think I am, cancer did not care... I was struck with triple negative breast cancer the first time in 2013. Triple negative affects young women and women of color. It is aggressive. Due to Black women not getting checked in a timely manner, we have a bigger risk of fatality with this disease. This takes me to my next and biggest point – it is imperative to listen to your body!

Get your mammograms between 40 and 49. Studies show that women who are between 50-79 are at the highest risk for breast cancer. I was 47 when I was first diagnosed, and then again at 49. My cancer was textbook: Triple negative will return in 18 months. And it did just that! The first round I did 13 units of chemo, dealing with the red devil, and it was just that – a devil. It took away my hair, skin, and gave me neuropathy in the feet and fingertips, but I never lost my dignity, fight, or faith in God!

I completed my treatment with 37 units of radiation. The second time, the doctor decided that I needed to have my breast removed. So I went through breast removal with full breast reconstruction. For a woman, this can be devastating.

Through all of this journey, I learned to depend on my family and loved ones...and most of all God! I realized that this was not about me, it was about God, and how I was going to react to the charge that I had been given. I decided to kick it into gear and take charge! It was just me and God! It was my children, and my family, it was my friends.

It took many prayers, and much love to get me through. Nothing in my life will ever be taken for granted. Life is a gift!

In closing I could sit and talk about the horrible things that happened in this journey, but I have chosen to live in the light! The bright light! Knowing that without my venturing down this ugly road called cancer, my life would not be as full and rich and lovely and peaceful. I would not know how to savor each day, how to love, and be loved, and how to venture and do whatever my heart tells me to do!

Thanking God each day for making me a CHAMPION!

From Keynon Lake

CEO/Founder of My Daddy Taught Me That,
Author, Public Speaker, Activist

I have been a lifelong friend of Mr. Joe Greene, and truly consider him a brother. While I have known him to have different jobs and take on several projects, his passion is truly uplifting, serving, and helping his community. From creating FUNNY'R'US, an avenue to provide laughter for his community, to being a pivotal figure in My Daddy Taught Me That, working with our youth, to now dedicating his life to getting as many people to go get tested for colon cancer – it would be an understatement to say that he cares.

To give context as to how much he cares, let me add this. While going to college seeking a higher education, Mr. Greene picked up a felony charge as a young man in life. We all know that to most folks, a felony charge can truly hurt you from advancing or moving forward. To me, having a felony is 10 times more problematic for a Black man living in this country. Through all his difficulties, setbacks, and hurdles, Mr. Greene did not waver.

Instead of taking the mindset of "I gotta get mine. I gotta push and grind for myself and my family," he chose to still push and grind for the people he supported and the ones who needed it most.

It has truly been an honor to see the growth of Mr. Greene, but more importantly knowing what he has been dealing with and is facing, words cannot express the strength and determination he exudes. Again I cannot say this loud enough: Mr. Greene, while facing this ordeal that would have the majority of us truly clinging to the life we have and doing whatever we can or want to make our lives better, Mr. Greene chose to do what he does – HELP PEOPLE.

I am humbled and honored to call this man my brother.

RESOURCES

Videos

What the Health, Kip Andersen and Keegan Kuhn, directors, available online at Netflix and through https://www.whatthehealthfilm.com

"Asheville Man Raises Colon Cancer Awareness with Early Screening," interview with Joe Greene on Spectrum News, https://spectrumlocalnews.com/nc/mountain/news/2021/10/11/raising-colon-cancer-awareness?cid=app_share

Book

Chris Wark, *Chris Beat Cancer,* Hay House Inc.; 2nd edition (January 5, 2021)

Articles

American Cancer Society. "Colorectal Cancer Rates Higher in African Americans, Rising in Younger People." September 3, 2020. Retrieved from: https://www.cancer.org/latest-news/colorectal-cancer-rates-higher-in-african-americans-rising-in-younger-people.html

American Cancer Society. "What is Colorectal Cancer?" Retrieved from: https://www.cancer.org/cancer/colon-rectal-cancer/about/what-is-colorectal-cancer.html

American Cancer Society. "Do I Have Colorectal Cancer? Signs, Symptoms and Work-Up." Retrieved from https://www.cancer.org/latest-news/signs-and-symptoms-of-colon-cancer.html

CDC. "What Are the Symptoms of Colorectal Cancer" Retrieved from: https://www.cdc.gov/cancer/colorectal/basic_info/symptoms.htm

Mayo Clinic. "Colon Cancer: Symptoms and Causes" Retrieved from: https://www.mayoclinic.org/diseases-conditions/colon-cancer/symptoms-causes/syc-20353669

NBC News. "Chadwick Boseman's Death Shed Light on Colon Cancer, but Rates Remain High Among Black People." August 28, 2021. Retrieved from: https://www.nbcnews.com/news/nbcblk/chadwick-bosemans-death-shed-light-colon-cancer-rates-remain-high-blac-rcna1795

Organizations

My Daddy Taught Me That, a nonprofit organization mentoring young men of color, "Where Our Father's Hand Shapes Tomorrow's Man," https://mydaddytaughtmethat.org

Project Access, through the Western Carolina Medical Society, providing medical care for low-income and uninsured residents of Western North Carolina, https://www.mywcms.org/what-we-do/for-patients-and-community/ (The very first Project Access began in Buncombe County, North Carolina in 1996 and has since spread to many other communities across the U.S.)

HERS LLC, an organization founded by Yvette Jives (Joe Greene's mother), providing counseling and support to help empower underinsured and uninsured people as they seek medical care, https://www.hersnc.org

ACKNOWLEDGMENTS

You don't realize you need a support system until they all show up for you. I want to thank my family and friends for being there with me. I am grateful for all my treatment teams, the doctors and staff, for all their hard work and commitment to my health. I especially thank my Mama for being right by my side through every appointment, and making sure I had someone with me every step of the way.

DIAGRAMS

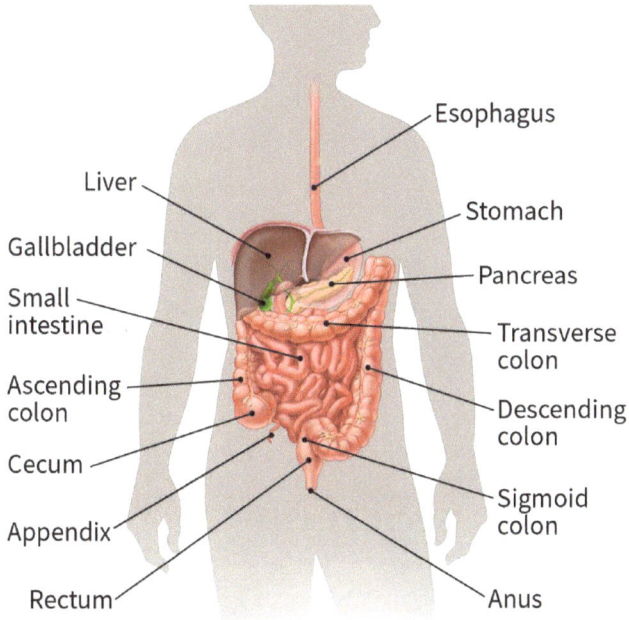

- Esophagus
- Liver
- Stomach
- Gallbladder
- Pancreas
- Small intestine
- Transverse colon
- Ascending colon
- Descending colon
- Cecum
- Sigmoid colon
- Appendix
- Anus
- Rectum

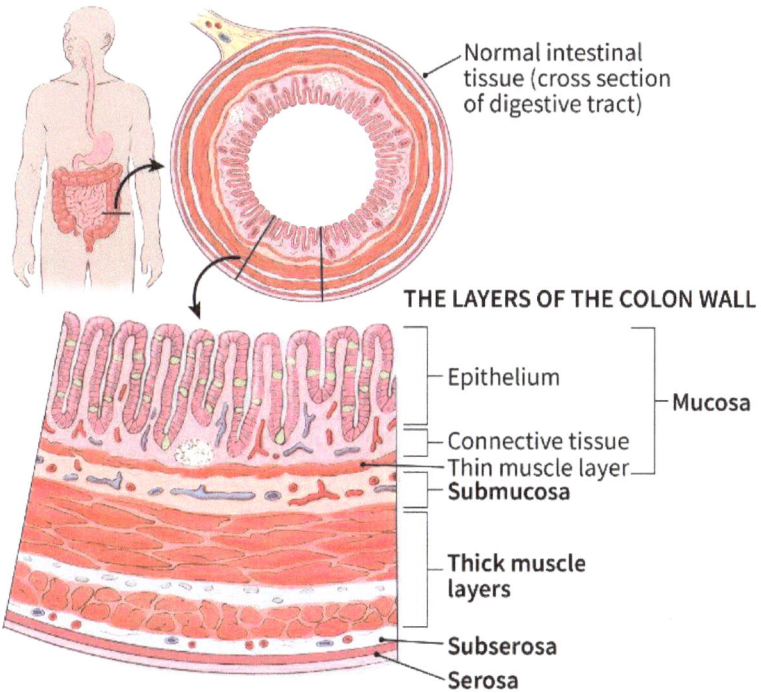

Normal intestinal tissue (cross section of digestive tract)

THE LAYERS OF THE COLON WALL

- Epithelium — Mucosa
- Connective tissue
- Thin muscle layer
- **Submucosa**
- **Thick muscle layers**
- **Subserosa**
- **Serosa**

ESSL

Early

Screening

Saves

Lives!!!

Visit the website:

www.ESSL2021.com

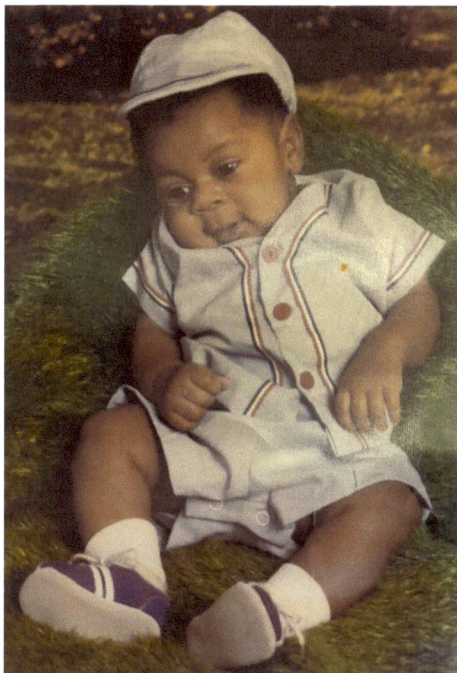

Just a cool guy...

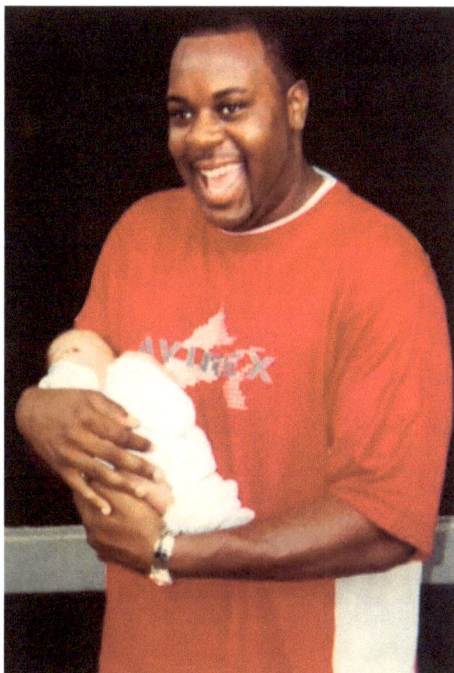

Young MJG (me) holding my nephew for the first time

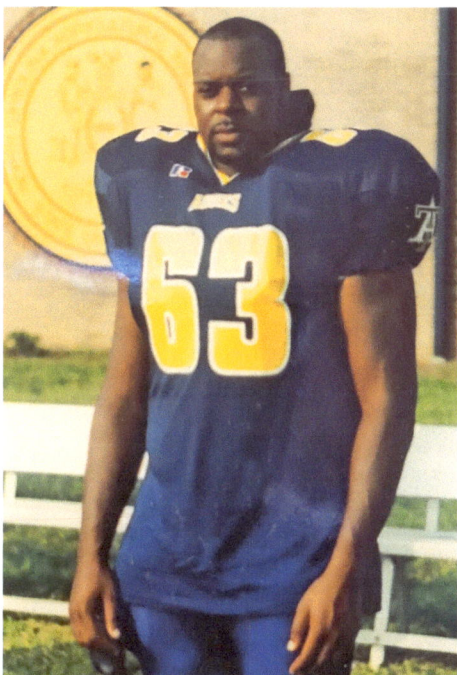

Starting offensive guard for NC A&T State University 2000-2001

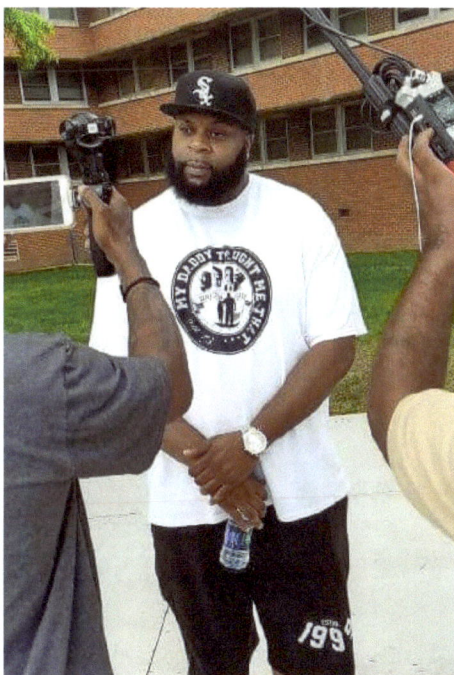

NC A&T (Cooper Hall)

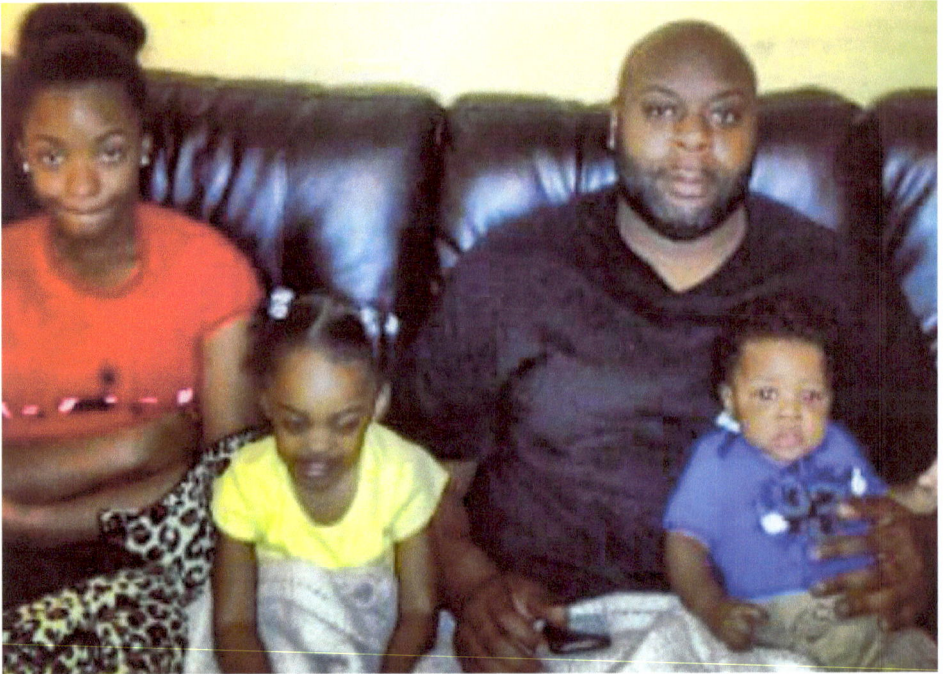

KJG ENTERPRISES . . . My kids

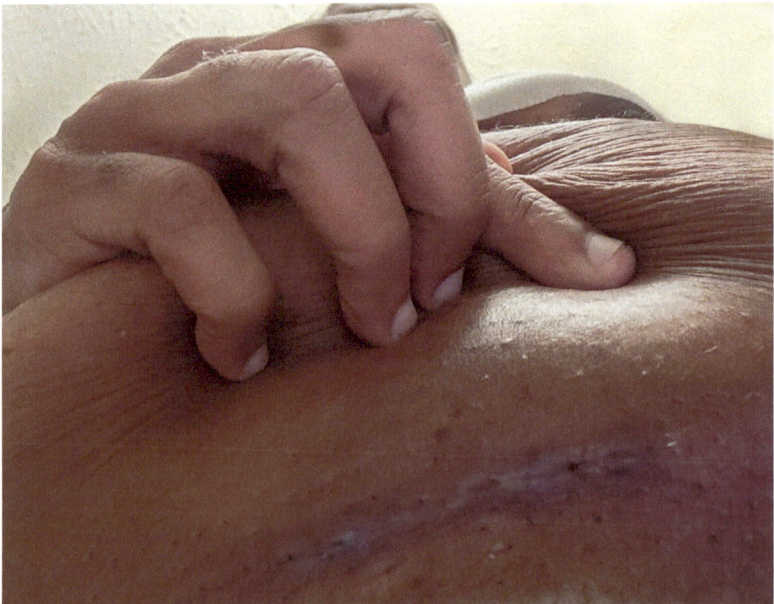

My C-section cut from surgery...where they took the mass of a tennis ball (the cancer) out of my colon

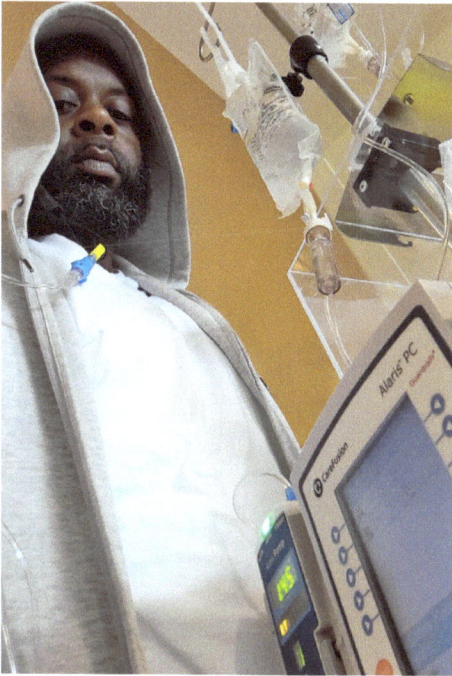

Chemo treatments...Each one a 4-5 hour process

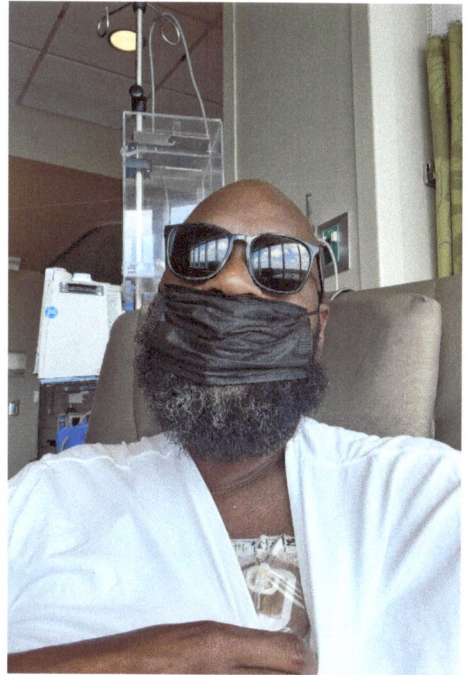

Just pushing through the BS...The taste and smells drive my mental crazy!!!!

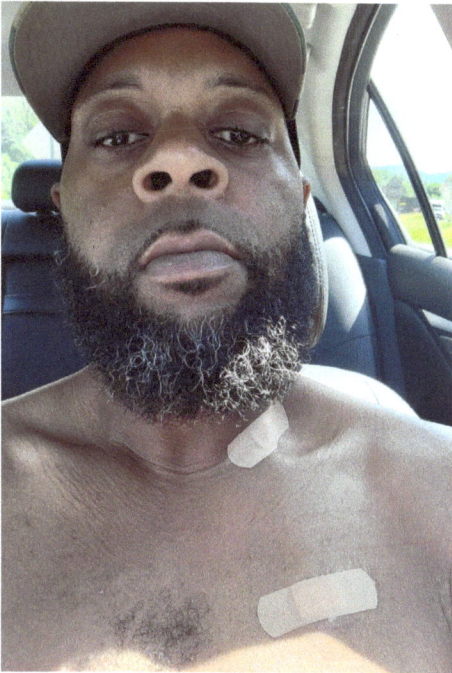

Took me months to keep bandaids off... couldn't look at the port pushing out of my chest

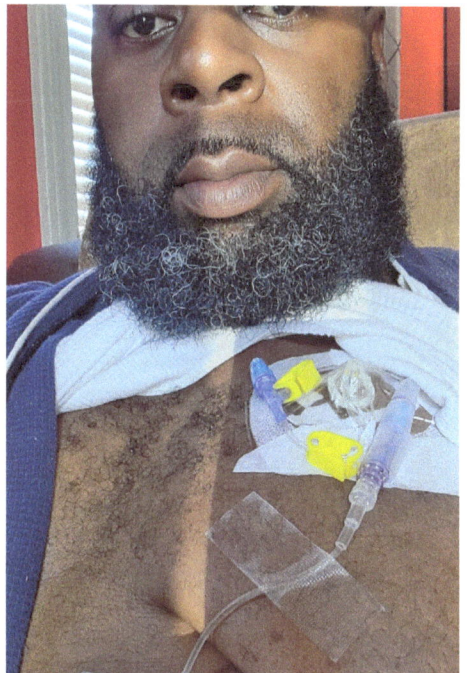

Home from chemo with a grenade-sized medicine ball attached to my port pumping 72 more hours of medicine

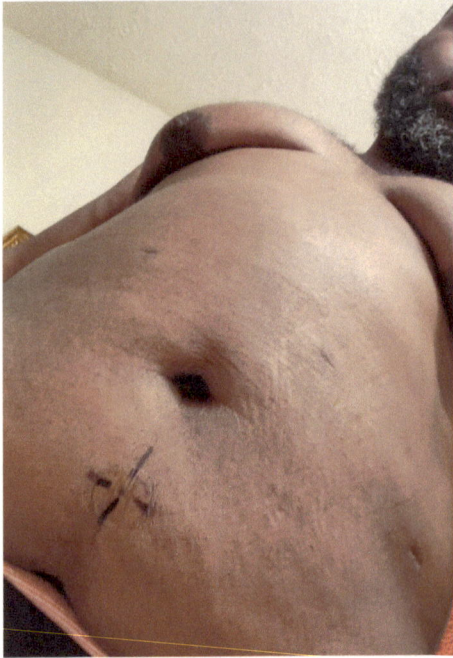

My scars...Emergency surgery cut 7 times and radiation tattoo to hit the exact spot every time in treatments

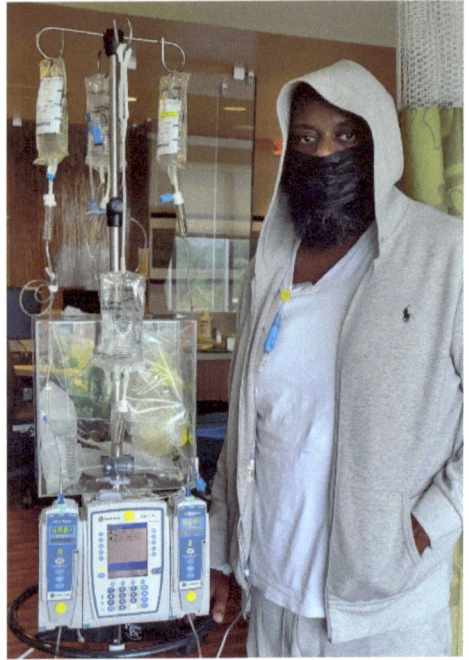

The second round of chemo...Much more intense than the first round and harder to manage

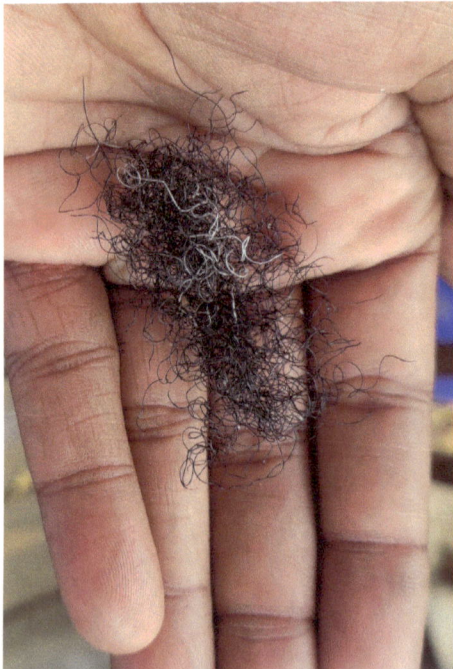

My beard coming out in clumps from chemo treatments

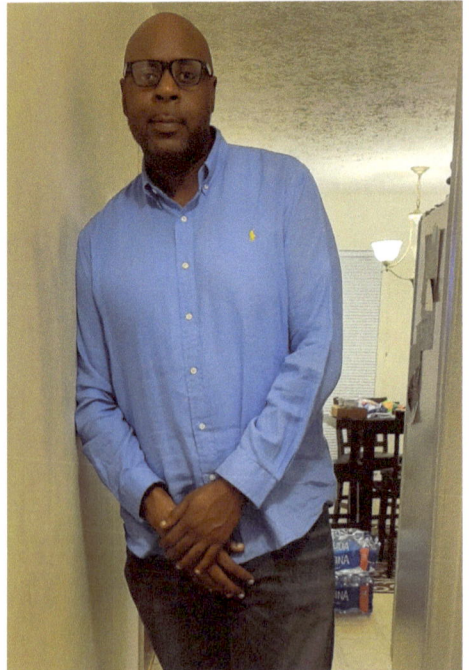

After all of my facial hair along with other parts of my body were affected by chemo treatments

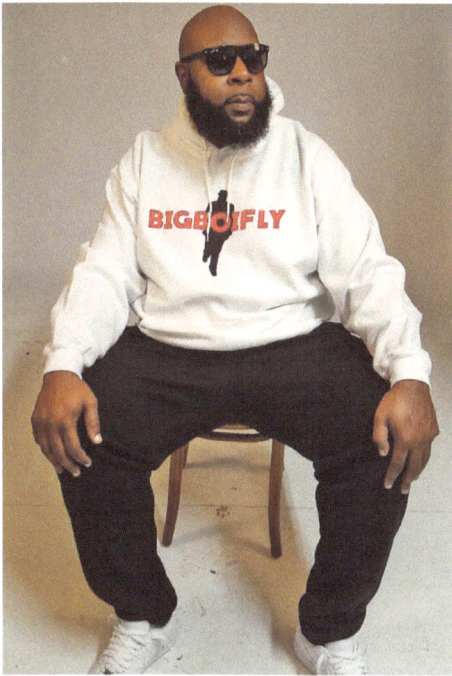

My clothing line...Made for big guys, originally BIGBOIFLY

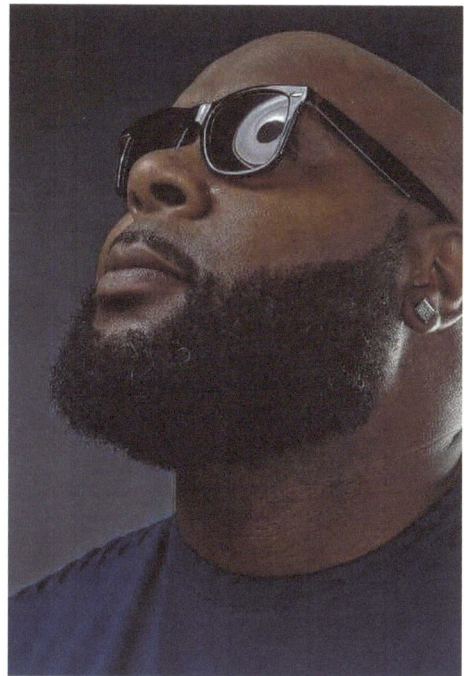

Head to the Sky...

For more information and to keep up with me,
check out my podcast SnappyNappyDugout
in support of Early Screening Saves Lives (ESSL)
and covering topics of interest to the community.

https://www.youtube.com/@snappynappydugout

SNAPPY
NAPPY
DUGOUT